Family Therapy Techniques

FAMILY THERAPY TECHNIQUES

Salvador Minuchin
H. Charles Fishman

Harvard University Press
Cambridge, Massachusetts, and London, England

Library of Congress Cataloging in Publication Data

Minuchin, Salvador.
  Family therapy techniques.

  Includes bibliographical references and indexes.
  1. Family psychotherapy.   I. Fishman, Herman
Charles, 1946–   joint author.   II. Title.
RC488.5.M56   616.89´156   80-25392
ISBN 0-674-29410-6

To the Philadelphia Child Guidance Clinic,
an institution that throughout its existence has
encouraged exploration and supported deviancy
in the search for better systems of caring for
children

Acknowledgments

This book began a number of years ago when H. Charles Fishman and Thomas A. Roesler, both students of Salvador Minuchin, proposed a book about how they were learning the techniques he taught. During the succeeding years, the book went through many transformations as the senior author's conceptualizations and ways of teaching changed.

We are grateful to Peggy Papp for her contribution of "The Greek Chorus and Other Techniques of Paradoxical Therapy," *Family Process* 19, no. 1 (March 1980), which is appearing as Chapter 16 of this book. Since paradoxical interventions are not a technique that we use as frequently as some schools of family therapy do, we are presenting her article as a clear statement on this subject.

We want to thank Dr. Roesler for his contributions to the early discussions of the book, and Dr. Patricia Minuchin for her suggestions and collaboration in the chapter on family development. We would also like to thank Virginia LaPlante for her editorial counsel, Marge Arnold for her tireless help, and as always, Fran Hitchcock, without whom the book would have been longer and poorer.

Contents

Family Therapy Techniques

1 Spontaneity

The word *techniques* implies craftsmanship: attention to detail, concern with the product's function, and investment in results. It brings images of a well-joined corner, a smooth-running drawer, the delicate mother-of-pearl inlays in a medieval doorway, the intricacy of Greek mosaics, or the harmonious filigree work of the Alhambra. But the phrase "techniques of family therapy" poses problems. It brings images of people manipulating other people. Specters of brainwashing, or control for the sake of personal power, hover. The moral concern is absolutely justified. Furthermore, technique alone does not ensure effectiveness. If the therapist becomes wedded to technique, remaining a craftsman, his contact with patients will be objective, detached, and clean, but also superficial, manipulative for the sake of personal power, and ultimately not highly effective.

Training in family therapy should therefore be a way of teaching techniques whose essence is to be mastered, then forgotten. After this book is read, it should be given away, or put in a forgotten corner. The therapist should be a healer: a human being concerned with engaging other human beings, therapeutically, around areas and issues that cause them pain, while always retaining great respect for their values, areas of strength, and esthetic preferences. The goal, in other words, is to transcend technique. Only a person who has mastered technique and then contrived to forget it can become an expert therapist. The effortless

1

jump of a Nijinsky is the product of years of careful study that have culminated in a control related to art, not technique.

What is the art of family therapy? It means to join a family, experiencing reality as the family members experience it, and becoming involved in the repeated interactions that form the family structure and shape the way people think and behave. It means to use that joining to become an agent of change who works within the constraints of the family system, intervening in ways that are possible only with this particular family, to produce a different, more productive way of living. It means to enter the labyrinth that is the family, and produce Ariadne's thread.

THERAPEUTIC SPONTANEITY

Family therapy requires the use of self. A family therapist cannot observe and probe from without. He must be a part of a system of interdependent people. In order to be effective as a member of this system, he must respond to circumstances according to the system's rules, while maintaining the widest possible use of self. This is what is meant by therapeutic spontaneity.

In common use, the word *spontaneity* suggests "unplanned." Therefore, "training for spontaneity" sounds like a contradiction in terms, a conclusion confirmed by the Webster's definition of spontaneity as "proceeding from natural feeling or native tendency without external constraint." But this difficulty is related to a cultural set. In modern times in Western culture, people are used to thinking of human beings as individuals independent of the constraints of context. As a result, they define *spontaneity* as sparsely as Australians define *snow*. Eskimos have several words for snow, describing the different varieties of the substance. So do skiers. But to Australians, who have never seen snow, much less tried to label its varieties, snow is merely *snow*. And that is how common usage defines *spontaneity*.

But when therapists look at human beings in their social context with an understanding of the constant interplay between person and context, the word *spontaneity* takes on richer meaning. It then comes closer to its root definition: "of its own motion (like a river following its course)." In this sense, a spontaneous therapist is a therapist who has been trained to use different aspects of self in response to different social contexts. The therapist can react, move, and probe with freedom, but only within the range that is tolerable in a given context. Like the term *dependency,* a nineteenth century pejorative which in the twentieth century has become a recognition of ecological fact, *spontaneity* gains richness in relation to context.

Study a de Kooning painting from close up. The individual strokes seem unrelated to each other, crossing and combining at random. Then move back and observe them from a distance. Now the women from Acabonig or the women from Sag Harbor appear on the canvas. The undulating line that seemed unrelated to the others is part of a woman's breast. Even in the most abstract of his paintings, after a while the lines begin to play with each other. Each line responds to the other lines, each organized in relation to the others. The painting, bounded by the frame, is a system of harmony, and each line relates to the whole.

The freedom of the painter is restricted by the first line on the canvas. Writers, too, know that their characters take on a life of their own, developing an autonomy that demands a particular unfolding. Pirandello's *Six Characters in Search of an Author* is a metaphoric statement about the demands a production makes on its author. Spontaneity, even the spontaneity of the mind, is always constrained by context.

The therapist's spontaneity is constrained by the context of therapy. The therapist, an influencer and changer of people, is inside the field that he is observing and influencing. His actions, though regulated by the goals of therapy, are the product of his relationship with the client family. The therapist is like the continuo player in a Baroque suite. He is free to do whatever feels right, as long as he remains within the harmonic structure. That is how things are.

But look at the advantages that contextual constraints bring to therapy. Because the therapist experiences the family reality, and because the rules of the family structure him from within the field, his interventions fall within a tolerable range. Interventions that are ineffective do not become chaotic or destructive; they are merely assimilated by the family without producing change. In a way, it is the constraints of the situation that give the therapist freedom. Because he is dependent on the field in which he is participating, his spontaneity is shaped by the field. Therefore, he can be comfortable in the knowledge that he does not have to be correct. In this situation, he will at least be approximate. He can allow himself to probe, knowing that at worst his responses will yield useful information. If he goes beyond the threshold of what is acceptable, the system will correct itself. He can be spontaneous precisely because he is reacting within a specific context.

The training of family therapists has similarities to the ancient training of samurai warriors. Miyamoto Musashi, a master samurai of the fifteenth century, described the techniques of survival in combat, some of which are startlingly close to the techniques of family therapy. He talked about "soaking in": "When you have come to grips and you are striving together with the enemy and you realize that you cannot advance, you 'soak in' and become one with the enemy . . . you can often win decisively with the advantage of knowing how to 'soak' into the enemy, whereas, were you to draw apart, you would lose the chance to win." When the samurai cannot see the enemy's position, he must "move the shade": "You indicate that you are about to attack strongly to discover his resources. It is easy then to defeat him with a different method once you see his resources."[1] Comparing these techniques with therapeutic joining shows that, although therapy is not a martial art, the therapist, like the samurai, must let himself be pulled and pushed by the system in order to experience its characteristics.

The training of the samurai, too, was a training for spontaneity. Only if the sword was a continuation of the arm could the samurai survive. The attention to detail that the samurai considered essential for achieving spontaneity was extraordinary. To become a master, he had to train as a warrior for three to five years. Then, having become a craftsman, he was required to abandon his craft and spend a number of years studying unrelated areas, like painting, poetry, or calligraphy. Only after achieving mastery in these different intellectual endeavors could a warrior go back and take up the sword, for only then had the sword become a continuation of the arm. He had become a samurai because he had forgotten technique. This, clearly, is the meaning given to the concept of the spontaneous therapist.

Technical expertise does not admit uncertainty; a skilled craftsman is certain of his craft. Therefore, a therapist invested in mastering techniques must guard against becoming too much the craftsman. He could become so enamored of his ability to join two pieces of beautiful wood that he failed to realize they were never supposed to join. Fortunately, the therapeutic system inhibits craftsmanship by pushing the therapist to experience and respond from within. Reality can be seen only from the perspective that the therapist has in the system. As a result, reality is always partial, and any truth a half-truth. Techniques so painstakingly learned must therefore be forgotten, so that, finally, the therapist can become a healer.

METHODS OF TRAINING

The spontaneous therapist has to have knowledge about the characteristics of families as systems, the process of their transformation, and the participation of the therapist in that process. These are theoretical constructs, which are learned deductively. The specific skills of therapy, on the contrary, are transmitted inductively, in an apprenticeship process. The therapist learns the small movements of therapy and uses these in a building block process in repeated sessions, under supervision. In time, he learns to generalize.

By these means, the therapist finds himself with two different sets of information. One is the dynamics of the human situation. The other is the specific operations of the therapeutic encounter. It is as though he had a list of words on the one hand, and an epic poem on the other. The training process must connect the two levels. The theoretical constructs must suggest the therapeutic goals and strategies, which in turn govern the therapist's small interventions. The methodology of teaching the difficult art of family therapy has to be harmonious with both the concepts and the practices taught.

The development of a spontaneous therapist rules out several popular methods of teaching and supervision. It does not make sense, for instance, to supervise a therapist by asking him to describe a session if he is unaware of being inducted into the family system. It seems ineffective to train a therapist by having him role-play his position in his family of origin at different stages of his life, if what he needs is to expand his style of contact and intervention so that he can accommodate to a variety of families. And it seems inadequate to require a therapist in training to change his position in his family of origin, when his goal is to become an expert in challenging a variety of diverse systems. Although all these techniques may be useful for the therapist as a person in understanding his position in his own family system and achieving insight into his own and his family's functioning, they are not necessary or sufficient to become a spontaneous therapist. For that purpose, inductive methods of teaching and working with families from the beginning of training are more effective.

Ideally, a small group of five to eight students is placed in the charge of a supervisory teacher. There must be available to them a sufficient number of treatment families to provide a variety of therapeutic experience, as well as additional teachers to provide input at a more generic, theoretical level. The training also requires specialized equipment: a library of videotapes of the work of experienced therapists, a room with a one-way mirror for live supervision, and a complete videotaping system to record the students' work for subsequent analysis.

There are two phases of training, one devoted to observation and the other to practice. In the first phase, the teachers demonstrate their therapeutic style in live sessions, which the students observe. While one teacher does family therapy before a one-way mirror, another teacher behind the mirror gives the students a running commentary on the movements of the therapist. In the process of observing an experienced therapist, the students often become discouraged. They feel that they will never achieve the degree of knowledge and level of skill that are necessary for this magic intervention. They begin to attribute to the expert therapist a native wisdom unrelated to training and skill. But the teacher behind the mirror encourages them to concentrate on techniques, teasing out the specific operations for discussion and analysis.

This kind of observation is intermingled with observation and analysis of the tapes of other master therapists conducting therapy in different situations. The goal is to emphasize the therapist as a specific instrument. Teachers and students need to rely on their best utilization of themselves. By observing the style of the experts, the students are encouraged to examine their own therapeutic style.

An observer of Salvador Minuchin learns to focus on my concern with bringing the family transactions into the room, my alternation between participation and observation, my way of unbalancing the system by supporting one family member against another, and my many types of response to family members' intrusion into each other's psychological space. In families that are too close, I artificially create boundaries between members by gestures, body postures, movement of chairs, or seating changes. My challenging maneuvers frequently include a supportive statement: a kick and a stroke are delivered simultaneously. My metaphors are concrete: "You are sometimes sixteen and sometimes four"; "Your father stole your voice"; "You have two left hands and ten thumbs." I ask a child and a parent to stand and see who is taller, or I compare the combined weight of the parents with the child's weight. I rarely remain in my chair for a whole session. I move closer when I want intimacy, kneel to reduce my size with children, or spring to my feet when I want to challenge or show indignation. These operations occur spontaneously; they represent my psychological fingerprint. My therapeutic maneuvers are based on a theoretical schema about families and family transformation, and on my own style of using myself. I am comfortable with pushing and being pushed by people, knowing that if both I and the family take risks within the constraints of the therapeutic system, we will find alternatives for change.

The other phase of training consists of both live and videotape supervision of the students conducting their own therapy sessions. The context of live supervision is the interviewing room with a one-way mirror. The teacher-supervisor and the student group watch one student as he works with a family. A telephone connects the two rooms, allowing direct communication between the trainee and the supervisor. As the student interviews, he knows that the supervisor will telephone if necessary. This kind of training assumes that the students are already professional mental health practitioners, such as psychologists, psychiatrists, social workers, nurses, or ministers. The training of nonprofessionals requires a different, more intense format.[2]

There are different levels of supervisory intervention. For example, if one family member is remaining silent and the student therapist is responding only to the more active family members, the student may receive a call suggesting that he activate the family member who is withdrawing from the session or showing restlessness. If the supervisee gets stuck in an operation, the supervisor may ask him to come behind the one-way mirror for a conference about what to do in the rest of the session. The supervisor may enter the therapy room and consult with the student on the spot, or may remain in the room for a kind of cotherapy transaction. These kinds of intervention can occur at any point in the training. As the student becomes more knowledgeable, however, the more direct forms of intervention may lessen, until the supervision remains at the level of discussion prior to or after the session.

This kind of supervision might suggest an experience of intrusiveness. But in fact the student therapist develops a comfortable dependence on the supervisor, relying on his help to finish a session appropriately or to work through difficult moments. The student knows the supervisor will get him out of trouble.

Behind the mirror, the rest of the group observe their colleague and discuss the session with the supervisor. Thus, while a beginning therapist works directly with one family, he also follows the therapy of several other families, learning the difficulties faced and solutions found by each of his colleagues in developing an effective style of intervention.

Live supervision is, by design, a special form of cotherapy. The responsibility for the outcome of the interview falls on both the student and the supervisor. This method has several advantages. Students can start doing therapy before they feel ready, with the supervisor's backup. Because the supervision occurs in a real situation, it focuses on the idiosyncracies of the session. Understanding the dynamics of the family and the therapeutic system becomes ground; managing the immediate therapeutic transactions is figure. Teacher, student, and observers are concerned with the small brushstrokes necessary for the successful handling of the hour. The student's accumulated experience of his own and his colleagues' sessions will eventually allow him to reach the critical point at which the specific movements of therapy generalize into a method.

Throughout training, every session is videotaped for subsequent review. The focus in this form of supervision shifts to the student therapist. Because the supervisor is no longer responsible for the family, the family recedes to become ground; the style of the therapist is now figure.

The tape can freeze any part of the session, enabling the student to select a segment and explain his therapeutic goals during that segment. The tape thus shows the relationship between intention and result, between goal and skills. From it emerges a profile of each student's style: his strengths and difficulties, the particular way in which he turns his therapeutic concepts into strategies, and the means by which these strategies are implemented. The supervisor then prescribes measures to expand the student's skills. Within his own style, the student may work to become less central, to shorten speeches, to activate or deflect conflict, to emphasize family strengths, and so on. The teacher relates the prescriptions as specifically as possible to the student's observed behavior. During the next live supervision, the student is evaluated with respect to his implementation of the changes proposed. Before the session, the supervisor reminds the student of his task. During the session, the supervisor intervenes to help the student implement the change.

To expand a therapist's style is a difficult task for both teacher and student, since the student may lose confidence in his automatic way of functioning and become overdependent on the teacher for direction. The student usually becomes a less skillful therapist during this transitional period, since he no longer relies on his habitual responses and does not yet have new ones.

Every therapist needs certain specific skills in order to achieve the goals of family transformation, but each therapist has a different way of using himself in implementing these techniques. Supervisors must be alert to the different characteristics of the student therapists as well as of the families. Some therapists are excellent leaders from a down position. These people encourage families to teach the therapist how things are done. Other therapists find it more comfortable to assume a position of leadership from a power base. They are good at being the expert and operating from somewhat outside the family system. Both possibilities are different ways of using oneself well; there is no one correct way of achieving leadership. Etymologically, the word *education* means a drawing out, and training in family therapy is in many ways an education.

It is essential that training start with an overview of theory and that theoretical seminars accompany both of its phases, thus enabling the student to integrate practice with theory. The student should not be a technician, but a therapist. For a number of years the authors thought that to reach this goal, and to avoid the dangers of "teaching to the head" that characterized most traditional training in psychotherapy, we should emphasize the "steps of the dance": the specifics of therapy. Through an inductive process the student, in "circles of decreasing uncertainty," would arrive at the "aha!" moment: the theory. Emphasis on the student's own style would give him an understanding of the self as an instrument of therapy, as well as an expansion of his style that would really be a widening of his own life repertory. And all of this would be accomplished without burdening the student with a load of theory that would slow him down at moments of therapeutic immediacy and act as a barrier to the process of joining with the family. Although we disagreed with Carl Whitaker's contention that what family therapy needed was nontheory, in effect we joined him and Jay Haley in their suspicion of "large doses of theory," particularly for the beginning therapist.

But twenty years of teaching have shown us that there has to be a middle ground. The field of family therapy is full of clinicians who change chairs à la Minuchin, give directions à la Haley, go primary process à la Whitaker, offer paradoxes in Italian, tie people with ropes à la Satir, add a pinch of ethics à la Nagy, encourage cathartic crying à la Paul, review a tape of the session with the family à la Alger, and sometimes manage to combine all of these methods in one session. Probably this salad of techniques, if condimented with wit, can produce an immediate salutary flight into health in some families. But this is not an easily reproducible feat, and it will fail in the hands of the average therapist.

Training, then, requires not only a set of clearly differentiated techniques but also a few umbrella concepts to give them meaning.

Unfortunately, the teaching of new skills often disorganizes a beginning student. As in any learning or relearning process, the student finds himself concentrating so much on the trees that he misses the forest. The goals of therapy lose focus, becoming ground, while the techniques become figure. As in the training of the samurai, the student needs a number of years to achieve expertise and many more to achieve spontaneity.

True training for wisdom would require the student to disengage from the techniques of therapy and engage with the difficulties of life. Too many young therapists go into healing without the life experience necessary to understand the problems with which they are intervening. Ideally, they should exclude from their caseload families who are at a developmental stage that they have not yet experienced themselves. If that is impossible, they should acknowledge their ignorance and ask the families to educate them in these matters.

But as the student therapist increases his practice and experience, he begins to find that he does certain things well. Eventually a disconnected cluster of skills becomes an integrated style that fits with his person. He begins to find that certain metaphors, once used effectively with a certain family, come back to him in similar situations with a very different family. He begins to recognize that beneath the superficial discontinuities of family transactions, there are many similarities. He begins to thread together operations that at first seemed diverse. He begins to ponder whether a mother asking a child questions that require only a yes or no is isomorphic with the father taking an adolescent's coat off. On the way to becoming wise, the therapist finds himself moving from observations of particular transactions to generalizations about structure. He develops ways of transforming his insights into operations that have the intensity necessary to reach the family members. In this process of achieving a wisdom beyond knowledge, the therapist discovers that he has a repertory of spontaneous operations. Now he can begin to learn for himself.

2 Families

There is a tendency for living things to join up, establish linkages, live inside each other, return to earlier arrangements, get along whenever possible. This is the way of the world.

Lewis Thomas

In human terms, joining up in order to "get along" usually means some sort of family group. The family is the natural context for both growth and healing, and it is the context that the family therapist will depend on for the actualization of therapeutic goals. The family is a natural group which over time has evolved patterns of interacting. These patterns make up the family structure, which governs the functioning of family members, delineating their range of behavior and facilitating their interaction. A viable form of family structure is needed to perform the family's essential tasks of supporting individuation while providing a sense of belonging.

Family members do not ordinarily experience themselves as part of this family structure. Every human being sees herself as a unit, a whole, interacting with other units. She knows that she affects other individuals' behavior, and that they affect hers. And as she interacts within her family, she experiences the family's mapping of the world. She knows that some territories are marked, "Do as you please." Others are marked, "Proceed with caution." Still others are marked, "Stop." If she

11

crosses this limit, the family member will encounter some regulatory mechanism. At times she will acquiesce; at other times she will challenge. There also are areas marked, "Entrance forbidden." The consequences of transgression in these areas carry the strongest affective components: guilt, anxiety, even banishment and damnation.

The individual family members thus know, at different levels of awareness and specificity, the geography of their territory. Each family member knows what is allowed, what counterdeviation forces there are, the nature and efficiency of the monitoring system. But because she is a lone voyager in the territory of the family and the larger world, the individual family member rarely experiences the family network as a gestalt.

To a family therapist, however, the network of family transactions appears in all its complexity. She sees the total that is greater than the sum of its parts. The family as a whole seems almost like a colony animal—that entity composed of different life forms, each part doing its own thing, but the whole forming a multibodied organism which is itself a life form.

It is difficult for a student to look at this multibodied animal that is the family. Indeed, it is difficult for anyone reared in Western culture to look beyond the individual. We are trained into both an ethical and an esthetic preference for individual self-determination. To think of the individual as a segment of a larger social and biological unit is distasteful at best. Perhaps this is why those who attempt to come to grips with man's interdependence often resort to mystical or holistic philosophies connecting man with the universe. It is less painful to conceive of man as part of a universal intelligence than as part of the family network, a living organism closer to our experience. We can embrace man the cosmic hero, but we would prefer to turn a blind eye to his fight with his wife over who should have locked the front door.

Yet we know that the football player on a team, or the oboist in a quintette, somehow take on the excellencies of these more-than-human units. We experience the impulse that makes a stadium crowd of thirty thousand rise and yell in unison. And in therapeutic terms, any clinician can provide vignettes of the workings of the multibodied animal known as the family. There is even reason to believe that family "connections" go beyond the behavioral level to the physiological. In research with psychosomatic families, Minuchin and others found evidence which suggests that in some families, at least, stress between parents can be measured in the bloodstream of their observing child.[1]

The student therapist does not have to accept the idea of a conjoined physiology. But she does have to look at the family as more than an aggregate of differentiated subsystems, as an organism in itself. For it is the family's pulse she will feel. She will experience its demands for accommodation, and will feel comfortable only when proceeding at its tempo. She will experience its threshold for the appropriate and the shameful, its tolerance for conflict, its sense of what is ridiculous or sacred, and its view of the world.

The problems of studying the family are exacerbated by Western languages, which have few words or even phrases for describing units of more than one. There is the term *symbiosis* to describe a two-person unit in circumstances that are pathologic in the extreme, where one of its members "feels totally as a part and has inadequate experience of himself as a whole," in Albert Scheflen's words, so that a psychotic episode may occur when there is a break of affiliation in the organism.[2] But this term ignores normal interactions. Although the mental health field has a vast array of studies of normal transactions between mother and child, it has no word to describe this complex two-person unit. One could coin a term, such as *mochild* or *chother,* but it would be impossible to devise terms for all the multiple units.

Arthur Koestler, addressing this conceptual difficulty, observed that "to get away from the traditional misuse of the words whole and part, one is compelled to operate with such awkward terms as 'sub-whole' or 'part-whole.'" He coined a new term "to designate those Janus-faced entities on the intermediate levels of any hierarchy": the word *holon,* from the Greek *holos* (whole) with the suffix *on* (as in pro*ton* or neu*tron*), which suggests a particle or part.[3]

Koestler's term is particularly valuable for family therapy, because the unit of intervention is always a holon. Every holon—the individual, the nuclear family, the extended family, and the community—is both a whole and a part, not more one than the other, not one rejecting or conflicting with the other. A holon exerts competitive energy for autonomy and self-preservation as a whole. It also carries integrative energy as a part. The nuclear family is a holon of the extended family, the extended family of the community, and so on. Each whole contains the part, and each part also contains the "program" that the whole imposes. Part and whole contain each other in a continuing, current, and ongoing process of communication and interrelationship.

THE INDIVIDUAL HOLON

To view the individual as a holon is especially difficult for anyone brought up in Western culture. Take the Census Bureau's definition of a nonfamily: "a single unattached adult." Here is a striking example of our individualistic ideology. Nowhere among living organisms can one find "unattachment," yet it exists in our human typologies. The Constitution, tax and social security laws, health delivery systems, mental health and education services—even those expensive residential homes for senior citizens only—all express not only the concept but the desirability of the autonomous individual.

This bias has permeated the mental health field, extending even into the field of family therapy. Ronald Laing's concept of family politics demands that the individual be freed from his noxious family shackles (probably facilitating his inclusion in the census tract as an unattached single adult). Murray Bowen's "differentiation of self scale," used to estimate the degree that the "self" remains uninfluenced by relationships, similarly highlights the "struggle" between the individual and the family. When the individual is seen as being part of any larger whole, somehow she is seen as losing out.[4]

The student therapist may be particularly prone to focus on the constraints the family imposes. The odds are high that she grew up in a family, where she struggled with the processes of individuating within the family group. It is also likely that she is at a stage in her own life cycle of separating from her family of origin and possibly forming a new nuclear family, where the demands of creating the new holon may be experienced as a challenge to her experience of self. The student may therefore have to focus rather conscientiously on the realities of interdependence and the workings of complementarity.

The individual holon incorporates the concept of self-in-context. It includes the personal and historical determinants of self. But it goes beyond them to include the current input of the social context. Specific transactions with other people elicit and reinforce those aspects of the individual's personality that are appropriate to the context. The individual, in turn, affects the other people, who interact with her in certain ways because her responses have elicited and reinforced their responses. There is a circular, continuous process of mutual affecting and reinforcing, which tends to maintain a fixed pattern. At the same time, both individual and context have the capacity for flexibility and change.

It is easy to view the family as a unit and to see the individual as a holon of that unit. But the individual includes other aspects that are not contained in the individual as a holon of the family, as shown here:

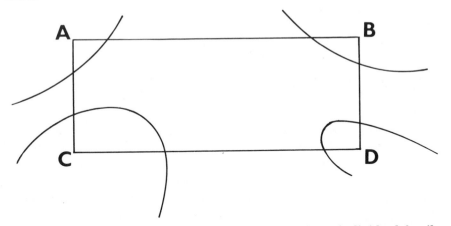

The rectangle represents the family. Each curve is an individual family member. Only certain segments of the self are included in the family organism. For *C* and *D* the family is more necessary than for *A* and *B*, who may be more related to colleagues, to their families of origin, and to peer groups. But the range of permitted behavior is still governed by a family organization. How wide a range of behavior can be included in the family program depends on the family's capacity to absorb and incorporate energy and information from the extrafamilial.

The constant interaction in different holons at different times requires the actualization of different segments of the self. A child interacting with her overinvolved mother operates with helplessness, to elicit nurturance. But with her older brother, she operates shrewdly and competitively, to get what she wants. A man who is an authoritarian husband and father within the family has to accept a lower hierarchical position in the world of work. A young adolescent, who is dominant in the peer group when in coalition with his older brother, learns to be polite when his brother is not there. Different contexts call forth different facets.

As a result, people are always functioning with a portion of their possibilities. There are many possibilities, only some of which are elicited or constrained by the contextual structure. Therefore, breaking or expanding contexts can allow new possibilities to emerge. The therapist, an expander of contexts, creates a context in which exploration of the unfamiliar is possible. She confirms family members and encourages them to experiment with behavior that has previously been constrained by the family system. As new possibilities emerge, the family organism becomes more complex and develops more acceptable alternatives for problem solving.

Families are highly complex multi-individual systems, but they are themselves subsystems of larger units—the extended family, the block, the society as a whole. Interaction with these larger holons produces a significant part of the family's problems and tasks as well as of its systems of support.

In addition, families have differentiated subsystems. Each individual is a subsystem, as are dyads, like husband and wife. Larger subgroupings are formed by generation (the sibling subsystem), gender (grandfather, father, and son), or task (the parental subsystem). People accommodate kaleidoscopically in these different subsystems. A son has to act like a child in the parental subsystem so that his father can act as an adult. But when he is left in charge of his younger brother, the child takes on executive powers. Within the family holon, three units in addition to the individual are of particular significance: the spouse, parental, and sibling subsystems.

THE SPOUSE HOLON

In family therapy it is useful to conceptualize the beginning of a family at the point in time when two adults, a man and a woman, join with the purpose of forming a family. This agreement does not have to be legal to be significant, and our limited clinical experience with homosexual couples with children suggests that family therapy concepts are as valid with them as with heterosexual couples with children. Each of the new partners has a set of values and expectations, both recognized and unconscious, ranging from the value of self-determination to whether people should eat breakfast. These two value sets must be reconciled over time to make a life in common possible. Each spouse has to give up part of his or her own ideas and preferences, losing individuality, but gaining belonging. In the process, a new system is formed.

The transactional patterns that slowly evolve usually are not recognized as such. They are simply there, part of the underpinnings of life, necessary, but not really thought about. Many have evolved with little or no effort. If both spouses come from patriarchal families, for instance, they may simply take it for granted that the woman will do the dishes.

Other transactional patterns are the result of stated agreement: "It's your turn to cook." In either case, the patterns established govern the way each spouse experiences self and partner in the spouse context. Eventually behavior that differs from what has become accustomed will hurt. Deviance will spark a sense of betrayal, even if neither partner has any conscious idea of what the trouble is. There will always be points of friction, and the system will have to adapt to meet changed contextual demands. But at some point, a structure underlying the spouse transactions will have evolved.

One of the spouse subsystem's most vital tasks is the development of boundaries that protect the spouses, giving them an area for the satisfaction of their own psychological needs without the intrusion of in-laws, children, and others. The adequacy of these boundaries is one of the most important aspects to the viability of the family structure.

If the nuclear family is seen apart from other contexts, each spouse appears to be the other's total adult context. In our extremely mobile society, the nuclear family can in fact be cut off from other systems of support, resulting in an overloading of the spouse subsystem. Margaret Mead cited this situation as one of the stresses endangering the family in the Western world. The spouse subsystem is therefore a powerful context for confirmation and disqualification.

The spouse subsystem may offer its members a supportive platform for dealing with the extrafamilial world, and it may provide them a haven from outside stresses. But if the rules of the subsystem are so rigid that the experiences gained by each spouse in extrafamilial transactions cannot be incorporated, the "spouses-in-the-system" may be bound to inadequate survival rules by past contracts and allowed a more diversified use of self only when away from each other. In this situation the spouse subsystem will grow more and more impoverished and devitalized, ultimately becoming unavailable as a source of growth for its members. If these conditions continue, the spouses may find it necessary to dismantle the system.

The spouse subsystem is vital for the child's growth. It is her model for intimate relationships, as expressed in daily interactions. In the spouse subsystem the child sees ways of expressing affection, of relating to a partner who is stressed, and of dealing with conflict as equals. What she sees will become part of the child's values and expectations as she comes in contact with the outside world.

If there is any major dysfunction within the spouse subsystem, this will reverberate throughout the family. In pathogenic situations, a child may be scapegoated, or possibly co-opted into an alliance with one spouse against the other. The therapist must be alert to the use of the child as a member in a subsystem to which she should not belong, as opposed to transactions that are legitimately related to the parental functions.

THE PARENTAL HOLON

Transactions within the parental holon involve the familiar child-rearing and socializing functions. But many other aspects of the child's development are also affected by her interactions within this subsystem. Here the child learns what to expect from people who have greater resources and strength. She learns to think of authority as rational, or as arbitrary. She learns whether her needs will be supported, and she learns the most effective ways of communicating what she wants within her own family's style. Her sense of adequacy is shaped by how her elders respond to her and by whether this response is age-appropriate. She learns which behaviors are rewarded and which are discouraged. Finally, within the parental subsystem, the child experiences her family's style of dealing with conflict and negotiation.

The parental holon can vary widely in composition. It may include a grandfather or an aunt. It may largely exclude one parent. It may include a parental child, who is delegated the authority to guard and discipline her siblings. The therapist will have to find out who the subsystem members are; it does little good to coach a mother if the child's real parent is her grandmother.

As the child grows and her needs change, the parental subsystem must change as well. As the child's capacity increases, she must be given more opportunities for decision making and self-control. Families with adolescent children should negotiate differently from families with younger children. Parents with older children should give more authority to the children while demanding more responsibility from them.

The adults in the parental subsystem have the responsibility to care for, protect, and socialize the children, but they also have rights. The parents have the right to make decisions that are related to the survival of the total system, in such matters as relocation, selection of schools, and the determination of rules that protect all family members. They have the right, and indeed the duty, to protect the privacy of the spouse subsystem and to determine what role the children will play in the family's functioning.

In our child-oriented culture, we tend to stress the obligations of the parents and pay less attention to their rights. But the subsystem that is given tasks must also have the authority to carry them out. And although a child must have the freedom to explore and grow, she will feel safe to explore only if she has the sense that her world is predictable.

Problems of control are endemic in the parental holon. They are continually being tackled and more or less resolved by trial and error in all families. The nature of the solutions will vary at different family developmental stages. When a family gets stuck in this area and comes to therapy, it is essential that the therapist pay attention to the participation of all members in the maintenance of the dysfunctional transaction and in the possible availability of resources for problem solving.

THE SIBLING HOLON

Siblings form a child's first peer group. Within this context, children support each other, enjoy, attack, scapegoat, and generally learn from each other. They develop their own transactional patterns for negotiating, cooperating, and competing. They learn how to make friends and deal with enemies, how to learn from others, and how to achieve recognition. They generally take different positions in the constant give and take, and the process furthers both their sense of belonging to a group and their sense of individual choices and alternatives within a system. These patterns will be significant as they move into extrafamilial peer groups, the classroom system, and later the world of work.

In large families the siblings organize themselves in a variety of subsystems according to developmental stages. It is important for the therapist to speak the language of different developmental stages and to be familiar with their different resources and needs. It is useful to create in the sibling context scenarios for the exercise of skills of conflict resolution in a number of areas, such as autonomy, competition, and competence, which may later be practiced in extrafamilial subsystems.

Family therapists tend to underutilize sibling contexts and overutilize therapeutic designs that demand an increase of parental diversity of functioning. But meeting with siblings alone, organizing therapeutic moments in which the siblings discuss certain issues while the parents observe, or developing "dialogs" between the sibling and parental holons can be extremely effective in creating new forms for resolving issues of autonomy and control. In divorced families, meetings between the siblings and the estranged parent are particularly useful as a mechanism to facilitate a better functioning of the complex "divorced organism."

How the family carries out its tasks is not nearly as important as how well. Family therapists, the product of their own culture, must therefore guard against imposing the models that are familiar to them, as well as the rules of functioning that are familiar. Family therapists must guard against a tendency to punctuate around the nuclear family, dismissing the significance of the extended family—its communication with and impact on the nuclear. Younger therapists may find themselves sympathetic with the rights of children, not having experienced the complexities of parenting. They may find themselves judging parents guilty without understanding their efforts. Male therapists may tend to unbalance the spouse subsystem, understanding and supporting the male spouse's position. Female therapists, concerned about the constraints imposed on women by a patriarchal family, may support the differentiation of the female spouse beyond the possibilities that exist in a particular family. Therapists must remember that families are holons imbedded in a larger culture, and that the therapist's function is to help them become more adequate within the possibilities that exist in their own family and cultural systems.

DEVELOPMENT AND CHANGE

The family is not a static entity. It is in the process of continuous change, as are its social contexts. To look at human beings apart from change and time is solely a construct of language. Therapists, in effect, stop time when they look at families, like stopping a motion picture to focus on one frame.

Yet family therapy has tended not to explore the fact that families change over time. This is partly because family therapists are intensely oriented to the here and now, as opposed to psychodynamic therapy's exploration of the past. But it is also owing to the fact that a family therapist experiences the family structure's governing power with enormous impact. She has entered a living system that has its own ways of being, and powerful mechanisms for preserving those ways. In the immediacy of the therapeutic encounter, these stabilizing mechanisms are what is felt; the flexible elements of the structure rarely impinge so strongly. Change is going on in the present, but it gains salience only in the long view.

The family is constantly subjected to demands for change, coming from within and without. A grandparent dies; the whole parental subsystem may need realignment. The mother is laid off from work; the spouse, executive, and parental subsystems may have to be modified. Change is, in fact, the norm, and a long-range view of any family would show great flexibility, constant fluctuation, and quite probably more disequilibrium than balance.

To look at a family from the long view is to see it as an organism evolving over time. Two individual "cells" join, forming a multibodied entity like the colony animal. This entity moves through stages of aging that affect each body individually, until the two progenitor cells decay and die, while others start the life cycle anew.

Like all living organisms, the family system has a tendency toward both maintenance and evolution. Demands for change may activate counterdeviation mechanisms, but the system evolves toward increasing complexity. Although the family can fluctuate only within a given range, it has an amazing capacity to adapt and change while maintaining continuity.

Living systems with these characteristics are by definition open systems, in contrast with the closed "equilibrium structures" described in classical thermodynamics. Ilya Prigogine explains the difference: "A crystal is a typical example of an equilibrium structure. Dissipative [living] structures have a quite different status: they are formed and maintained through the effect of exchange of energy and matter in nonequilibrium conditions." In a living system, fluctuations, occurring either internally or externally, take the system to a new structure: "a new structure is always the result of an instability. It originates from a fluctuation. Whereas a fluctuation is normally followed by a response that brings the system back to the unperturbed state, on the contrary, at the point of formation of a new structure, fluctuations are amplified." Classical thermodynamics, Prigogine concludes, "is essentially a theory of destruction of structure ... But in some way such a theory has to be completed by a theory of creation of structure."[5]

For years family therapy emphasized the power of systems to maintain themselves. Now the work of Prigogine and others has shown that if a system is partially open to the inflow of energy or information, "the ensuing instabilities do not lead to random behavior ... instead, they tend to drive the system to a new dynamic regime which corresponds to a new state of complexity."[6]

The family, a living system, exchanges information and energy with the outside. Fluctuation, either internal or external, is normally followed by a response that returns the system to its steady state. But when the fluctuation amplifies, the family may enter a crisis in which transformation results in a different level of functioning that makes coping possible.

This view of the family as a living system suggests that the long-range study of any family would show the following development, in which periods of disequilibrium alternate with periods of homeostasis, and the fluctuation remains within a manageable range:

This model gives the therapist a base for moving quickly to the relationship between family developmental stage and therapeutic goals, because the therapeutic crisis follows a developmental blueprint. Unlike other models, this one is not limited to individual and context. It deals with holons, postulating that developmental changes in the individual affect the family, and that changes in the family and extrafamilial holons affect the individual holons.

Family development, according to the model, moves in stages that follow a progression of increasing complexity. There are periods of balance and adaptation, characterized by the mastery of appropriate tasks and skills. There are also periods of disequilibrium, which arise from either the individual or context. These result in a jump to a new and more complex stage, in which new tasks and skills are developed.

Consider a two-year-old who is sent to nursery school. Experimenting with new coping skills away from her mother, she begins to demand new relationships within the family. The mother, counting to ten in the crowded grocery store, has to allow her to select the school's brand of cookies. That evening the father has to comfort the mother with a joke about the "terrible two's." The truth is that all three of these family members must outgrow the stage of infant/parent-of-infant. The child, the mother-child dyad, and the family triad are in a dissipative structure. Fluctuation has amplified because of both internal and external inputs, and the ensuing instabilities will move the system to a new complexity.

The developmental model posits four main stages, organized around the growth of children. These include couple formation, families with young children, families with school-age or adolescent children, and families with grown children.

COUPLE FORMATION

In the first stage, the transactional patterns that form the structure of the spouse holon are developed. The boundaries that govern the relationship of the new unit to the families of origin, to friends, to the world of work, and to the neighborhood and other significant contexts must be negotiated. The couple must work out new patterns of relating to others. They must maintain important contacts, while also establishing a holon whose boundaries are clear enough to permit the growth of an intimate couple relationship. Questions arise constantly. How often will they visit his twin sister? How do they resolve his dislike of her best friend? What do they do about the late hours at the lab that are part of her professional dream, but which leave him eating alone twice a week?

Within the spouse holon, the couple will have to reconcile their different styles and expectations and develop their own ways of processing information, relating, and dealing with affect. They must develop rules about closeness, hierarchies, areas of specialization and expertise, and patterns of cooperation. Each has to develop the ability to sense the other's vibes, evolving common associations and shared values, hearing what is important to the other, and reaching some agreement about how to handle the fact that they do not share all values.

Above all, the spouse holon must learn to deal with conflict, which occurs inevitably when two people are forming a new unit—whether the issue is closed or open windows in the bedroom at night or the family budget. The development of viable patterns for expressing and resolving conflict is a crucial part of this early period.

This stage is clearly a dissipative one. There is a high degree of information exchange both between holon and context and within the holon itself. There is also tension between the needs of the couple holon and the needs of its individual members. Rules that were previously satisfactory to each individual alone must be modified.

In the formation of a couple, the issues of part and whole are highly significant. Each spouse at first experiences him or herself as a whole interacting with another whole. In forming the new couple unit, each must become a part. This can be felt as a ceding of individuality. In some cases the therapist working with a family at this stage may have to focus on complementarity, to help the couple realize that belonging is enriching as well as constraining.

As time goes by, the new organism will stabilize as a balanced system. This evolution to a higher level of complexity is anything but painless. But if the holon survives at all, the couple will reach a stage where, in the absence of significant internal change or external input, the system's fluctuations will remain within the established range.

FAMILIES WITH YOUNG CHILDREN

The second stage occurs with the birth of the first child, when new holons are instantly established: parental, mother-child, father-child. The spouse holon must reorganize to deal with new tasks, and new rules must be developed. The newborn is totally dependent on responsible care. At the same time, the newborn is demonstrating elements of her own personality, to which the family must accommodate.

This is another dissipative structure—to the point that the system itself may be endangered. The wife may be caught in conflicting demands for her time and loyalty. The husband may move for disengagement. A therapist may have to move the father toward the mother and child, reengaging him in parental functions and helping him to build a more complex, differentiated view of himself in the spouse and parental holons.

If these problems are poorly resolved, cross-generational coalitions may form. The mother or father may unite with the child in a coalition against the spouse, keeping him peripheral or making him overcontrol.

While dealing continually with issues of control and socialization, the family must also negotiate new contacts with the external world. Relationships to grandparents, aunts and uncles, and cousins are formed. The family must cope with hospitals, schools, and the whole child-industry of clothing, food, and toys.

As the child begins to move around and talk, the parents must establish controls that give them space while maintaining safety and the parental authority. Adults who have established patterns of nurturance must now modify those patterns, developing appropriate methods of maintaining control while encouraging growth. New patterns must be explored and stabilized in all family holons.

As other children are born, the stable patterns established around the first child are disrupted. A more complex and differentiated family map, including a sibling holon, must develop.

FAMILIES WITH SCHOOL-AGE OR ADOLESCENT CHILDREN

A sharp change occurs when children go off to school, initiating the third developmental stage. Now the family must relate to a new, well-organized, highly significant system. The entire family must develop new patterns: how to help with school work and who should help; what rules to enforce about bedtime, homework, and leisure; and how to encompass the school's evaluation of their child.

As the children grow, they bring new elements into the family system. The child learns that her friends' families operate by different, and patently fairer, rules. The family will have to negotiate adjustments, changing some rules. The new boundaries between parent and child must permit contact, while freeing the child to reserve certain experiences to herself.

With adolescence, the peer group gains strong power. This is a culture in itself, with its own values about sex, drugs, alcohol, dress, politics, life style, and the future. Now the family is interacting with a strong and often competing system, and the adolescent's increasing competence makes her better able to demand accommodation from her parents. Issues of autonomy and control must be renegotiated on all levels.

The children are not the only family members who are growing and changing. There are specific passages in adult life, which tend to center around decades. These stages, too, affect and are affected by the family holons.

At this stage, another source of pressure and demand may begin to impinge on the family: the parents' parents. Just when middle-aged parents are dealing with questions of autonomy and support with their growing children, they may have to negotiate a re-entry into their own parents' lives, to compensate for declining strength or bereavement.

A minor imbalance requiring adaptation is characteristic of families through much of this third stage. But dissipative conditions are evident at the time of school entrance and at various points in adolescence when sexual needs, school demands, and the competing appeals of the peer group disrupt the established patterns in the family.

Finally, the process of separation begins at this stage, and this change resonates throughout the family. A second child may have had a relatively disengaged position within an enmeshed parental holon. But when her older sister goes off to college, she finds herself under increasing parental scrutiny. The tendency to recreate accustomed structures by drawing a new member into the previously established pattern is great. When this happens, it may represent a failure in adapting to the demands of family change.

FAMILIES WITH GROWN CHILDREN

In the fourth and final stage the children, now young adults, have formed their own commitments to a style of life, a career, friends, and ultimately a partner. The original family is once again a family of two. Although now the family members have a long history of changing patterns together, this new stage requires a clear reorganization around how parents and children will relate to each other as adults.

This is sometimes called the "empty nest" period, a term conventionally associated with the depression of a woman whose occupation is gone. But what is actually happening is that the spouse subsystem, once again, becomes the crucial family holon for both partners, although if there are grandchildren, these new relationships will have to be worked out. This period, often described as a period of loss, can instead be a period of great development if the spouses, both as individuals and as a couple, draw on their accumulated experiences, dreams, and expectations to realize possibilities that were unattainable while parenting was necessary.

This developmental schema describes only the middle-class family, with husband, wife, and 2.2 children. More and more, it is likely that the family will also form some sort of extended network or will experience divorce, desertion, or remarriage. In moving through such stages, people also face very complicated challenges. But whatever the circumstances, the basic flow remains: a family has to go through certain stages of growth and aging. It must cope with periods of crisis and transition.

What is significant for therapy is the fact that both change and continuity are the way of any living system. The family organism, like the individual human, moves between two poles. One pole represents the security of the known. The other is the exploration necessary for adaptation to changing conditions.

When a family comes to treatment, it is in difficulty because it is stuck in the homeostatic phase. Demands for the status quo constrain the family members' ability to deal creatively with changed circumstances. Adherence to rules that were once more or less functional handicaps the response to change. One of the goals of therapy is, therefore, to move the family to a stage of creative turmoil where what was given must be replaced by a search for new ways. Flexibility must be induced by increasing the system's fluctuations, ultimately moving it toward a higher level of complexity. In this sense, therapy is an art that imitates life. Normal family development includes fluctuation, periods of crisis, and resolution at a higher level of complexity. Therapy is the process of taking a family who are stuck along the developmental spiral and creating a crisis that will push the family in the direction of their own evolution.

3 Joining

The family therapist must, from the beginning, take some sort of leadership position. Theoretically, family and therapist enter therapy with the same goals. The family's presence is an acknowledgment that they want help and that they are inviting the therapist, an expert, to enter their system and help them change a situation that is maintaining or producing stress, discomfort, or pain. In practice, however, the family members and the therapist may, and usually do, differ in their understanding of the location of the pain, its cause, and the process of healing.

The family has generally identified one member as the location of the problem. They think the cause is that individual's internalized pathology. They expect the therapist to concentrate on that individual, working to change him. To the family therapist, however, the identified patient is only the symptom bearer; the cause of the problem is dysfunctional family transactions; and the process of healing will involve changing those dysfunctional family transactions. Fluctuation will have to be amplified to move the family system toward a more complex form of organization—one that copes better with the current family circumstances.

Consequently, the therapist's input may activate the mechanisms within the family system that preserve its homeostasis. During the family's common history, rules that define the relationships of family members to one another have developed. Any challenge to these rules will be countered automatically. Furthermore, a family coming to therapy has been struggling to resolve the problems that brought them for some time. Their attempts to cope may have narrowed their life experience. They tend to overfocus on the problem area, and because they are under stress, they tend to overutilize familiar responses. Family members thus have less freedom than usual, and their capacity for exploration has been reduced.

So family and therapist form a partnership, with a common goal that is more or less formulated: to free the family symptom bearer of symptoms, to reduce conflict and stress for the whole family, and to learn new ways of coping. Two social systems have joined, for a specific purpose and for a certain time.

Now the functions of the participants in the therapeutic system must be defined. The therapist is in the same boat with the family, but he must be the helmsman. What are the characteristics of that helmsman? What qualifications must he have? What implicit or explicit map of these waters can he use to guide the craft?

The therapist does not yet know the idiosyncrasies of this particular family dance, but he has seen many family dances. He also has his own genetic coding and his own life experience. He brings an idiosyncratic style of contacting, and a theoretical set. The family will have to accommodate to this package, in some fashion or another, and the therapist will have to accommodate to them.

In most cases the family will accept the therapist as leader of this partnership. Nevertheless, he will have to earn his right to lead. Like every leader, he will have to accommodate, seduce, submit, support, direct, suggest, and follow in order to lead. But the therapist who has been trained in spontaneity can feel comfortable in accepting the paradoxical job of leading a system of which he is a member. He has developed some skill in using himself as an instrument of transactional change. He also has a body of knowledge and experience with families, systems, and the processes of change. He knows that by becoming a member of the therapeutic system, he will be subjected to its demands. He will be channeled into traveling certain roads in certain ways at certain times. Sometimes he will be aware of the channeling; other times he will not even recognize it. He must accept the fact that he will be buffeted by the implicit demands that organize the family members' behavior. He will tend to talk to the central member of the family, and smile secretly at the incompetence of the "schlemiel." He will feel the impulse to save the symptom bearer, or help in scapegoating him. His job as a healer requires him to be able to join the family in this way. But he must also have the skills to disjoin, then rejoin in a differentiated way—and there's the rub.

THERAPIST'S USE OF SELF

There is disagreement within the field of family therapy on precisely how a therapist uses himself to achieve the leadership of the therapeutic system. Early theories of therapy portrayed the therapist as an objective data gatherer, but this myth has largely been discredited. Even in psychoanalysis, the understanding of the analyst's use of self in the process of countertransference has sparked great changes in psychoanalytic theory and practice. "It is probably true," Donald Meltzer writes, "that any analysis which really taps the passions of the patient does the same for the analyst and promotes a development which can further his own self analysis." The necessary state for inspired interpretation is "that type of internal companionship which promulgates an atmosphere of adventure in which comradeship develops between the adult part of the patient's personality and the analyst as creative scientist . . . implying therapeutic possibilities for both parties to the adventure."[1]

Family therapists often acknowledge only the traditional views of the psychodynamic approach to therapy. It is interesting, therefore, to note how closely our concern with understanding the therapist's use of self is paralleled in the different paradigm of psychoanalysis.

When therapists began to see the family as a whole, their focus in studying the therapist's use of self was the danger that the therapist might be inducted into the family field to such a degree that he would lose therapeutic maneuverability. Lyman Wynne and others have described the confusion and anxiety therapists experience when working with schizophrenic families.[2]

Carl Whitaker's solution to the problem of maintaining therapeutic leverage is to have a cotherapist: "I don't think one therapist alone possesses the amount of power necessary to get in and change the family and get back out again . . . I don't want to stay the rest of my life with my finger stuck in the dike." With a cotherapist, the therapist can then solve his "countertransference problem by retreating into his relationship to the other therapist, and the therapeutic process then becomes a process of the two groups relating to each other." Whitaker trusts the "we," his cotherapist and himself, while not always trusting either of them alone; together they have "stereoscopic vision."[3] With the protection of the cotherapist, Whitaker, whose goal is a creative expansion for the family and for himself, enters into an intense personal involvement with the family, accepting the family impact on the therapist as inevitable and frequently beneficial.

At the opposite extreme is the Milano school, which postulates that induction is inevitable whenever the therapist engages closely with the family.[4] To avoid induction, the therapists involve themselves with their own group, composed of two cotherapists observed and supported by two other members of the team. The relationship between the therapists and family, while overtly a friendly one, is covertly an adversary relationship. The therapists design their interventions to produce resistance in the family, which in turn will produce behavior that the therapists consider therapeutic. The danger that the therapists will join with the family system and get caught in subsystem conflicts is avoided with extreme care.

Somewhere toward the middle of this continuum is Murray Bowen, who maintains his objectivity and controls his use of self by acting as a coach. The therapist in this position of expert is extremely central: he is the person to whom all communications are directed. People are encouraged to talk about emotional processes rather than experiencing them in the session. The therapist strives to maintain an emotionally calm atmosphere. What results is a therapeutic system quite dissimilar from, and less intense than, the natural family transactions. The diluted rules have only limited power to induct the therapist. Central but protected, the therapist conducts the session very much on his own terms.[5]

The authors' position on the therapist's use of self is that he must become comfortable with different levels of involvement. Any technique may be useful, depending on the therapist, the family, and the moment. At times the therapist will want to disengage from the family, prescribing like a Milano expert, perhaps with a hidden agenda to his program. At other times he will take a median position, coaching à la Bowen. At other times he will throw himself into the fray à la Whitaker, taking one member's place in the system, allying strongly with a family underdog, or using whatever tactic fits his therapeutic goal and his reading of the family. There are limitations on his use of self, determined by his personal characteristics and the characteristics of the family. But within these limits, the therapist can learn to use techniques that require different levels of involvement.

Joining a family is more an attitude than a technique, and it is the umbrella under which all therapeutic transactions occur. Joining is letting the family know that the therapist understands them and is working with and for them. Only under his protection can the family have the security to explore alternatives, try the unusual, and change. Joining is the glue that holds the therapeutic system together.

How does a therapist join a family? Like the family members, the therapist is "more human than otherwise," in Harry Stack Sullivan's phrase.[6] Somewhere inside, he has resonating chords that can respond to any human frequency. In forming the therapeutic system, aspects of himself that facilitate the building of common ground with the family members will be elicited. And the therapist will deliberately activate self-segments that are congruent with the family. But he will join in a way that leaves him free to jar the family members. He will accommodate to the family, but he will also require the family to accommodate to him.

The process of joining in a therapeutic system goes beyond simply supporting a family. Although joining is often related to supportive maneuvers, at other times it is effected by challenges to dysfunctional maneuvers which give the family the hope that the therapist can indeed make matters better. When a therapist like Whitaker works with families with psychotic members, he frequently enters the system with the demand that the family members accommodate to him. This "immovable object" technique is a powerful joining maneuver, combining the therapist's worldview, his understanding of the family process, and his self-respect. Although the technique can be quite startling for observers, it frames the therapeutic system in a way that conveys the possibility of help.

Since the therapist's use of himself in the therapeutic system is the most powerful tool in the process of changing families, he needs to be knowledgeable about the range of his joining repertory. It will not do for a therapist who is young and has a caressing voice to join like an indignant parent, as Minuchin sometimes does. It is important that the therapist should use his resources well, not that he should imitate the successful expert well. Another rule of thumb for successful joining is to work with families whose stage of development the therapist has experienced. If he must work with situations that he has not experienced, joining from a down position by asking for help in understanding them would be a good joining maneuver, since it gives time for the therapeutic system and the therapist to grow.

Like all human creations, joining is not necessarily a reasoned, deliberate process. Much of the joining process occurs beneath the surface, in the normal processes of people relating to people. It is also true that the therapist's own style will be compatible with some families, with whom he will find he can be very much himself. But in other families he may find himself acting more boisterous than usual, or more proper. With some families he will find himself being more verbal. With others, he will talk less. His rhythm of speech will change. With some families he will find himself talking more to the mother. In others, he will talk to all family members. He should observe the changes in himself as responses to the family's implicit transactional patterns and should use these external signals as another level of information about the family.

The therapist can join families from different positions of proximity. Specific techniques of joining are adapted to a close position, a median position, and a disengaged one.

CLOSE POSITION

In a position of proximity, the therapist can affiliate with family members, perhaps even entering into coalition with some members against others. Probably the most useful tool of affiliation is confirmation. The therapist validates the reality of holons he joins. He searches out positives and makes a point of recognizing and rewarding them. He also identifies areas of pain, difficulty, or stress and acknowledges that, although he will not avoid them, he will respond to them with sensitivity.

The therapist may confirm even family members he dislikes, and he need not study the methods of Pollyanna to do so. When people like someone, they program themselves to attend to facets of that person which confirm their view. The same process happens when they dislike people: they scan for negatives while ignoring positives. They shield themselves from uncertainty by focusing on those facets of a person or group that confirm them in their own position. The structural family therapist, knowing how people select observations in order to reinforce their beliefs, can direct himself to notice positives. After all, people coming for therapy are doing their best, as are we all.

In confirming what is positive about people, the therapist becomes a source of self-esteem to the family members. Furthermore, other family members see the confirmed person in a new light. The therapist increases his own leverage by establishing himself as a source of the family's self-esteem and status. He also amasses the power to withdraw his approval if the clients do not follow his lead.

Often confirmation is simply a sympathetic response to a family member's affective presentation of self, such as, "You seem to be concerned . . . depressed . . . angry . . . tired . . . washed out." Confirmation can also be a nonjudgmental description of a transaction among family members, such as, "You seem to be engaged in a continuous struggle," or, "When you talk, he disagrees . . . grows silent . . . feels challenged." This type of intervention is not an interpretation. The family members already know what the therapist is telling them. His statement is simply an acknowledgment that he has gotten the message and is willing to work with them on the problem.

Another way of confirming is to describe an obviously negative characteristic of a family member while at the same time "absolving" that person of responsibility for the behavior. To a child, the therapist might say: "You seem to be quite childish. How did your parents manage to keep you so young?" To an adult, the therapist could say: "You act very dependent on your spouse. What does she do to keep you incompetent?" In these techniques, the family member feels recognized in an area of difficulty without being criticized or made guilty about it, and he may respond to the therapist as if personally confirmed.

Confirmation goes on throughout therapy. The therapist continually scans for and emphasizes positive ways of looking at the family members' functioning while pursuing the goals of structural change. The therapist is always a source of support and nurturance as well as the leader and director of the therapeutic system.

When working in proximity, the therapist must know that his freedom of movement is being handicapped by his induction into the family system. By functioning in proximity, he achieves intensity. But he is also a participant caught in the rules of participation. It is important for the therapist to be able to use himself in this modality, but it is also essential for him to know how to disengage, after he has entered.

MEDIAN POSITION

In the median position, the therapist joins as an active, neutral listener. He helps people tell their story. This modality of joining, which is called tracking, is drilled into a therapist by the objective schools of dynamic therapy. It is a useful way of gathering data. But it is never as neutral and objective as the users think it is. And it too can hamper the therapist's freedom of movement. If family members are avidly telling their story, the therapist's attention may be locked into content. Sometimes a therapist tracks the communication of the most verbal family members, unaware of the family life being enacted before his unseeing eyes.

Working in the median range, the therapist can also tune into the family process. If the mother is the family switchboard and the father is peripheral, the therapist may join the family first by listening respectfully to the mother, even though his ultimate goal is to increase the father's power in the family.

The therapist can gather useful information about the family by observing his own way of tracking family process. Does he find himself talking mostly to the mother? Has he neglected to ask why the father did not come to the session? Does he find himself feeling protective toward one family member, or does he sense one family member as an irritant? The therapist, observing the pressures organizing his behavior, may join by choosing to yield to those pressures. He does not interpret his reactions to the family, since to do so would emphasize his role as an outsider, alien to the family. But he notes them to himself, both as a means of avoiding induction and as a means of becoming familiar with the structure that governs the behavior of this system's members.

The Javits family provides an example of tracking. The family came to treatment because the husband, the identified patient, was depressed. This exchange occurs in the middle of the first interview.

Minuchin (*to mother*): Do you think your house is too much of a mess?
Mother: My house is not much of a mess, but it could be better.
Minuchin: When your husband thinks the house is a mess, does he think that you are not a good manager?

The therapist tracks concretely, asking, in essence, "What effect does your behavior have on your husband's view of you?"

Mother: Yes.
Father: Yes.
Minuchin (*to mother*): And can he tell you that, or does he need to swallow it?

The tracking includes an inference about the transactional pattern between the spouses and leads the couple to an interpersonal exploration.

Mother: It varies—sometimes he can just blurt it out without its bothering him, and other times he keeps it in because I get upset when he brings it out. It depends on whether he can cope with my being upset at that time or not.

Father: I think when something like that irritates me, it builds up and I hold it in until some little thing will trigger it, and then I'll be very, very critical and get angry. Then I'll tell her that I just don't understand why this has to be this way. But then I try to be very careful not to be unreasonable or too harsh because when I'm harsh, I feel guilty about it.

Minuchin: So, sometimes the family feels like a trap.

Father: It's not the family so much; it's just—(*Indicates wife.*)

Tracking condenses the details of the husband's criticism into one metaphoric statement, a "trap," which has a higher affective intensity than feels comfortable to the mother. It forces the husband to a confrontation with the wife.

Minuchin (completing husband's gesture): Kit?

This simple tracking transforms a nonverbal statement into a verbal one.

Father (looking at wife): No, not her either. It's just the things she doesn't do versus the things she does in terms of how she spends her time. Sometimes I think her priorities should be changed.

Therapist: Kit, he is soft-pedaling my statement.

The therapist tracks process, or the affective difference between the first and second statements by the husband, and invites the wife to comment on the therapist's description of the husband's behavior.

Mother: About being trapped?

Minuchin: Yes, about being trapped. I think people sometimes get depressed when they are, like your husband, unable to be direct. He's not a straight talker. There's a tremendous amount of indirection in your family, because you are essentially very good people who are very concerned not to hurt one another. And you need to tell white lies a lot.

The therapist tracks by confirmation, focusing on the husband's depression in a descriptive, nonjudgmental fashion and framing a dysfunctional transaction as mutual protection.

Father: It isn't so much lying as it is not saying something that should be said.

Minuchin (to mother): And you do the same thing for him.

Mother: I'm indirect?

Minuchin: Ask him?

The therapist, after joining, is in a position in which he can unjoin, by asking the family members to transact with each other around the same issue.

Mother (to husband): Am I?

Father: I don't really know. Sometimes you seem very direct, but I find myself wondering if you are telling me everything about what's bothering you. You know, if you seem upset, I'm not always sure that I know what's bugging you.

Mother: That I can be upset for something like that because it wouldn't upset you?

Father: Maybe that's part of it.

Mother (smiling, but at the same time her eyes are watering): Because you always seem to know better than I do what is really upsetting me, what my problem is at that moment.

Minuchin (to father): You see what's happening now? She's talking straight, but she's afraid that if she talks straight, you will be hurt, so she begins to cry and she begins to smile. So she's saying, "Don't take my straight talk seriously, because it is just the product of a person who is under stress." And that's the kind of thing you do to each other. So you cannot change too much. Because you don't tell each other in what direction to change.

The therapist moves the level of transaction from content to interpersonal process, keeping the focus on the same issue. Here the therapist is clearly leading the spouse subsystem toward a therapeutic exploration.

Father: We don't argue much.

Mother: No, we don't.

Father: Because when we argue, I take a position I can defend logically, and that makes her feel helpless.

Mother: And I cry, and he feels helpless.

Minuchin: I want you to work on this. It's possible that if he can learn to be more critical, then he doesn't need to be depressed. And it's possible that if you can be more critical, you won't need to cry so much. Maybe then you can give each other more freedom. If you can tell him the things that bug you and he can hear it, maybe he can tell you that he wants the house to be less of a mess.

The therapist finally takes control of the therapeutic system by restructuring the intervention, suggesting alternative possibilities.

This session shows the complexity of the tracking maneuvers. Tracking means not only to follow but also gently to direct explorations of new behavior. It means to shift levels of tracking from content, to process, and to tie process concretely to content. Through coaching and gentle pushing, the therapist helps the family look at their transactions in a new way in an atmosphere of acceptance. The tracking maneuvers are supported by confirmation techniques in which stressful transactions are described as caused by caring. The therapist's restructuring interventions are also a part of joining, since they carry an element of hope in their description of alternative behavior.

Tracking demands a knowledge of the language that family members use. Tracking young children's communications requires from the therapist the skills of a polyglot. He needs to recognize the different language that, say, a two- or four-year-old uses, and to speak it himself with the child in the presence of the adults in such a way that he communicates also with them.

The Kuehn family is composed of the father and mother in their early thirties, and two daughters—Patti, who is four years old, and Mimi, who is two. The older daughter is the identified patient. Her presenting problem is that she is "uncontrollable." In the initial interview, after the parents have introduced themselves, the therapist talks with the identified patient.

Minuchin: Hello, How are you?

Patti: Fine. Can we play with toys?

Minuchin: We're going to get some toys. (*Kneels.*) You said that your name is Patti?

Father: Yeah.

Minuchin: Patti, what's the name of your sister?

Patti: Mimi.

Minuchin: Mimi? (*Puts his thumb in his mouth like Mimi and engages her little finger with his.*) Hello, Mimi.

Patti: Don't pick her up. Don't pick her up. Don't pick her up. Do you know why?

Minuchin: Why?

Patti: 'Cause she has a sore arm.

Minuchin: She has a what?

Patti: She has a sore arm because she fell out of her crib.

Minuchin (pointing): Which arm—this one, or this one?

Patti: Which one Mommy?

Mother: The left one. Which one is that?

Patti (pointing): This one, right?

Mother: Um-hum.

Patti: This one. She cracked her—ah— (*Looks at mother.*)

Mother: Collar bone.

Patti: Collar bone.

Minuchin: Oh, my goodness!

Patti: It went ka-bam! Do you know why? She fell out of her port-a-crib again.

Minuchin (to parents): Let's share that ashtray, so we need to sit together.

Father: Okay.

The therapist uses two maneuvers here that are important when one works with small children. One maneuver is related to size. The therapist kneels in order to be at the same height as the child with whom he is talking. The other maneuver is related to the appropriate level of language. Talking with four-year-old Patti, the therapist is concrete in his communication, asking her name and the name of her sister, and then pointing to both of Mimi's arms in his request for information. By questioning Patti, he assigns her a competent position as the person who responds and the older member of the sibling subsystem. With the two-year-old, his communication is at the motoric level. He says hello by hooking his finger to the girl's, putting his thumb in his mouth to mimic the girl, and making facial expressions that she mimics.

In joining this family with very young children, the therapist starts the session by establishing contact through the children. This is contrary to an approach used with families of school-age and older children, where the therapist would start by establishing contact with the executive subsystem. In families with preschoolers, it is possible for the therapist to contact the family in a playful, nonverbal language. This strategy introduces a relaxation, because the therapist presents himself as an authority who plays with children and contacts the adults as parents.

DISENGAGED POSITION

The therapist can also join with a family from a disengaged position. Now he uses his stance as an expert, creating therapeutic contexts that bring family members a sense of competence, or hope for change. He functions not as an actor, but as a director. Perceiving the patterns of the family dance, the therapist creates scenarios, facilitating the enactment of familiar movements or introducing novelty by forcing family members to engage with each other in unusual transactions. These techniques are change producing, but they are also methods of joining which increase the therapist's leadership, since he is experienced as the arbiter of the session's rules.

As an expert, the therapist monitors the family's worldview. He accepts and supports some family values and myths. Others he avoids or deliberately ignores. He learns how family members frame their experience that "We are the Smith family; we should behave in such a fashion." He pays attention to the communicational patterns that express and support the family experience, and he extracts the phrases that are meaningful to this family. He can use these phrases as a joining maneuver either to support the family reality or to construct an expanded worldview that will allow flexibility and change.

PROBLEMS

It may happen that a therapist needs to work with people whom he cannot easily join because they have a different value system or political ideology or different styles of contacting or just simply a different chemistry. If the therapist is in a situation in which he can refer the patient to a colleague whom he considers a better match for the family, that is the best solution. But frequently this is not possible, and the therapist may find that he becomes more challenging and less effective. The result of his interventions may be more confrontation and a sense of helplessness shared by both family and therapist.

The therapist should then remind himself that it is simply impossible for this family to be absolutely devoid of qualities that he shares. It may be difficult to find them, but they have to be there. The problem is just that the therapist is not sufficiently motivated to look for them.

Minuchin once referred to a colleague a family whose young adult son was a drug addict. The identified patient was dependent, selfish, self-indulgent, irresponsible—the list could go on and on—and he elicited in my colleague helpless controlling responses. In a short consultation at some point, I asked the therapist if he knew that this patient was a very good poet. He was startled by the realization that he could not conceive this possibility.

Whenever a therapist can be helpful to a patient, he also likes that patient, so the trick is to find a way to be helpful. If the therapist solves that problem just once, the difficulty in joining will disappear.

Joining with a child abuse family presents a particularly difficult problem. The therapist's immediate response may well be to side with the battered child, communicating his sense of outrage to the adults responsible. The same problem occurs with families who are psychologically abusing their children, restricting their development, or expecting behavior inappropriate to the child's developmental level. But in order to change the situation, the therapist must join with the system as a whole. The parents, too, must feel his support, as he will need their cooperation to work with the family. Finally, it behooves the therapist to look carefully at the role that the injured member plays in the maintenance of the system as a whole.

The Morris family consists of a mother, father, and eight-year-old son. The family was referred from a children's hospital because the parents abused their child. On one occasion they beat the boy so badly that he required hospitalization. As the mother speaks, the boy is sitting slightly outside the family circle. He is crying and looking at the floor.

Mother: Johnny is impossible to manage! He absolutely ruined Christmas for me and my husband.

Minuchin (to mother): It must have been terrible for you to have your Christmas ruined. How did your son do that?

The therapist is forcing himself to act against his own inclinations. It would give the therapist great pleasure at this point to tell the mother exactly what he thinks of people who mistreat children. But if this child is not to be removed from his parents—which is always a chancy solution—family change is his best hope. In order to achieve that change, the therapist must keep the family in therapy. This can be done only by creating a therapeutic system in which the parents feel supported and understood before there is any challenge. Furthermore, for the therapist to support the child at the beginning would leave the boy even more vulnerable to abuse. Whatever course therapy may eventually take, the first step is to join with the family experience, tracking their perception of the problem and sympathizing with them over their ruined Christmas.

Chronic disputes displayed in an embattled dyad present special problems in joining, especially before the therapist has achieved a leadership position in the therapeutic system. To take sides is to alienate the other person; to take neither side creates the risk of letting the conflict continue out of control, increasing the conflicting members' sense of hopelessness.

If he can, the therapist may take a distant position and wait until the storm subsides. But sometimes he will have to plunge into an unbalancing technique, joining with one member against the other, and hoping that it will not keep the family from coming again to the next session. In another situation, he may decide that the best strategy of joining is to challenge both members' behavior on the grounds that better functioning has to be possible.

In the first session with an embattled couple, the therapist may say, "You are right," to the wife and, to a promptly irate husband, "You are right as well." Then he continues, "But the payment for being right and righteous is to maintain a miserable life together." While not a soft joining maneuver, this challenge ("a pox on both your houses") conveys the therapist's sense of commitment to the couple.

A CASE EXAMPLE

The Bates family is composed of father, mother, and Bud, age 14, Bud's two sisters, ages 28 and 24, having married and left home. Bud is truanting, smoking pot, and feeling depressed. He was admitted to the day hospital, but he arrives late each morning, saying that he cannot motivate himself. The next session is conducted as a consultation.

Minuchin: The hospital invited me to meet with you to see if I can be of help. So I will be available to you for this next hour. Can some of you begin to tell me what are the issues that you have at this point?

The therapist begins by taking the stance of an expert. He invites the family to use his expertise: "I will be available to you for this next hour."

Mother: Our big problem right now, as it was when we came here, is Bud's reluctance to get out of bed in the morning, to be where he's supposed to be. Right now he should be here at nine-thirty in the morning. It isn't just getting him out of bed for clinic, it's for anything that he has to do. When he was going to regular school, he wouldn't get up.

Minuchin: Tell me, Bud, are you a night person? Do you stay up late?

Bud: Twelve or twelve-thirty.

Minuchin: Un-huh, so it's easier for you to be awake at night. You know, there are people who are morning people and there are people who are late people. You would say that you are more of a night person. You are more alive, more awake, more ready to do things in the evening?

When the mother plunges into a description of Bud's problem, the therapist interrupts her by turning to the identified patient. Because this does not follow the normal rules of courtesy, it is perceived as the action of an authority. His statement to Bud normalizes the problem: "You are more of a night person."

Bud: Not real late. It's just in the morning that I don't feel like doing anything.

Minuchin: But that means that you feel more active in the evening.

Bud: No, I feel active all day, but—

Minuchin: If you had a good alarm clock, that would solve it?

Bud: Well, the alarm clock I've got now—

Minuchin: Who is the alarm clock?

Bud: Well, I've got one of my own.

Minuchin: Do you have an alarm clock, or is mother an alarm clock?

Joining Bud by tracking what he is saying and normalizing the problem, the therapist shifts gears, introducing a metaphor of proximity, which implies that proximity is linked to the symptom. The therapist has noticed that Bud is sitting close to his mother, and they are exchanging various nonverbal signals. Humorously, and very gently, he challenges the mother-son holon.

Bud: I've got one.

Mother: And I've got one.

Minuchin: Are you certain she's not an alarm clock, Bud?

Bud: Yes.

Minuchin: Who wakes you up?

Bud: She does most of the time.

Minuchin: So, she's your alarm clock.
Mother: If you want to call it that.
Minuchin: Okay, so you have a function. You are an alarm clock!

In a light, bantering fashion, the therapist confirms the mother and tracks Bud. At the same time, her relationship to her son is called into question.

Mother: Well, at the present time, we have two alarm clocks in his bedroom—
Minuchin: And they don't work?
Mother: And me.

The mother joins the therapist.

Minuchin: That means, maybe, you could put on a third alarm, staggered, like one at seven-thirty, one at seven-forty, one at seven-fifty.
Mother: That's how I work it now.
Minuchin: My goodness! You must be a very deep sleeper, Bud.
Bud: Yeah.
Minuchin: I got up today at four o'clock in the morning. I couldn't sleep. I wish I could get your symptom. If your three alarm clocks don't work, you can sleep until twelve o'clock, one o'clock, two o'clock— what's the latest that you have been able to keep sleeping?
(*Bud looks at mother.*) Don't ask her. That is not her function. She's an alarm clock. Is she also a memory bank?

The therapist, who is an incurable storyteller, interprets the symptom as a good thing by commenting on his own insomnia. He also begins to monitor the proximity of mother and son. Joining and restructuring are moving rather fast in this segment because the therapist's own sense of comfort tells him that he is in the permissible range. So far the session has focused on concrete behavior and on small transactions the family feels comfortable with. Now the therapist contacts the silent father.

Minuchin: I bet you wish you had that capacity. When do you wake up?
Father: Me? Quarter to five, five o'clock. (*Looks at wife.*)
Mother (*nodding*): Yeah.
Father: Five o'clock.

Minuchin: Five o'clock in the morning? Is your wife the memory bank in the family? Because not only did Bud look at her for information, but you also just looked at her.

The therapist, joining all three family members, is already creating a focus that will organize the rest of the session. The content is daily life, and the tone is as light as a chat about the weather. Nevertheless, to the family, the therapist is a sorcerer: he is an expert who understands them.

Father: Yeah.

Minuchin: She is a very busy person. She is an alarm clock and a memory bank. (*To father.*) When do you go to work?

Father: I leave about a quarter to six, six o'clock.

Minuchin: What's your shift?

Father: Sometimes six, sometimes seven to four-thirty, five-thirty. It could be any time around the clock.

Minuchin: You work ten hours then?

Father: Sometimes ten, sometimes eleven, sometimes eight. Most of the time it's nine.

Minuchin: Does that give you overtime?

Father: Yeah.

Minuchin: So, when you work ten hours, you are pleased then because you have a couple of hours overtime. What kind of work do you do?

Father: I am a foreman in an electronics shop. We do circuits, printing.

Minuchin: That means you must have been working there for many years to become a foreman.

Father: Thirty years.

Minuchin: Thirty years! How old are you now?

Father: Fifty.

Minuchin: You started at twenty and you worked all the time in one job?

Father: Um-hum.

Minuchin: So you certainly have seniority at this point.

Father: Yeah.

Minuchin: How many people are in the shop?

Father: Seventeen.

Minuchin: And how many foremen?

Father: Two, but the other foreman has not been there quite as long as me.

Minuchin: So, you are secure in that job.
Father: Oh, yeah.

The therapist tracks the father, getting neutral information from him by asking concrete questions to maintain contact. Now the therapist will make a conceptual jump, connecting the information with the son's symptom.

Minuchin: So, we have a person like you who knows about time, and knows about schedules, and knows about responsibility. You have worked all your life?
Father: Um-hum.
Minuchin: How is it you got a kid that doesn't know about time, doesn't know about schedules, doesn't know about motivation? How did you manage this?
Father: I don't know. That's what we can't figure out.
Minuchin: Something failed.
Father: Yeah.

The therapist and father have joined in their interest in the father's work. Now the therapist connects the symptom to the father's failure in modeling. But his formulation is that "something"—not someone—failed. The father agrees immediately; he and the therapist are partners in a goal-directed activity.

Minuchin: Maybe you gave him the wrong model. Maybe he doesn't want to be like you.
Father: Could be.
Minuchin: Maybe he feels you work too hard and—what do you think? (*To Bud.*) You don't want to be like Father?
Bud: Yeah, I'd like to be like him.
Minuchin: To work thirty years in the same job, always from six to four, would you like that?
Bud: Yeah.
Minuchin: Most young people like you look at the old man and say, "That's not the life for me." You really would like to be like him?
Bud: Yes, I want to work in the same place he does.
Minuchin: You would like to work in the same place? Have you been there with him?
Bud: Yeah. (*Mother nods agreement.*)

Minuchin: You see, not only do you look at Mother and you activate her, but even when you don't look at Mother, she activates herself. (*Everyone laughs.*) I asked you, and you said, "Yes," and she said, "Yes." You know, she's wired to you people. (*To Mother.*) Are you so wired that if he answers, you say it?

Mother: I guess so, yeah.

The therapist has been tracking content when suddenly a small, nonverbal transaction provides data that support his focus, and he shifts back to a metaphor of proximity. The "wiring" metaphor is not one that the therapist normally uses; its selection here is related to the father's job, and it indicates that the therapist is accommodating to the family language.

Minuchin: Extraordinary! Isn't that wonderful, with families, how they get wired?

Father: That's true.

Minuchin: Great! That means that Bud did not look at Mother. I know, because you were looking at me. Beautiful. So there are some invisible wires that run from you to Mom. You can hear vibes?

Mother: Um-hum.

The therapist's description of overinvolvement is presented as an extraordinary feat and something positive a family organism is able to accomplish.

Minuchin: Have you always been like that, wired to people?

Mother: Well, I guess so, yeah. Because I've always been responsible for people.

Minuchin: So, you two are very responsible people, really. You (*to father*) are very responsible to your job, and you (*to mother*) are very responsible to the family. Is that the way in which you divide the work? Your responsibility is to provide for the family, and your responsibility is to care for the kids?

The therapist confirms both parents, emphasizing positives. Nevertheless, he is preparing to use the behavior he has just praised as a field of challenge.

Mother: Yeah.

Father: Um-hum.

Minuchin: And this has worked?

Mother: Up to this point, fine.

Minuchin: How many years have you been married?

Mother: We were married thirty years, and we have two other children besides Bud—two married daughters.

Minuchin (to Bud): You are the only boy in the family, and you are the youngest. How old are your other sisters?

Bud: Oh, Lana's about twenty—I don't know if it's twenty-five—(*Bud looks at father, but mother supplies the answer.*)

Mother: Twenty-eight and twenty-four.

Minuchin (to Bud): You operate both of them! Very good. Now that was beautiful, because Bud looked at Dad and activated him, and Mother activated herself. Beautiful. Very invisible, but very strong wires. So, twenty-eight and twenty-four. Your younger sister is really much older than you are. How long will you be the baby? Until you are 50? Or until you are 20? I don't know, some families keep babies for a long time.

Again, humor challenges the enmeshment while supporting the family member. The challenge is possible because this family feels quite comfortable with the light, bantering mood. By now, therapist and family seem to have been friends for years.

Bud: I don't know.

Minuchin: Ask your mother how long you will be the baby.

Bud: How long?

Mother: Until you grow up.

Minuchin: Ah, that can be a lifetime. You can be 70 years old and still be the baby. You know, check to see what she means by that. How long will that take? Check up. You know, mothers have special arithmetic. Check up with your mother about what is her arithmetic. How long will you be the baby?

Mother: How long will you be the baby? Until you accept responsibilities, which I'm willing to give you, but you have to accept them. And when you accept the responsibility for yourself, then I would consider you grown.

Minuchin (to Bud): Do you agree with that? It is only up to you to grow up?

Bud: Why are you putting all the responsibility on me?

Mother: Because it's your life. I am willing to guide, but I would like you to assume the responsibility.

Minuchin: Bud, I know people who are wired like your mom is to you—so closely wired that you don't get too much space. In other families, people who are wired as you are wired keep young for a long time.

Twenty minutes into the session, the therapist and family are connected and working at therapy together. In the rest of the session, the therapist elects to focus on the father. He explains that he is concerned about the mother: she is too ready to be available to people, and that cannot be good for her. She is too wired to others; the father must provide the wire cutters that will rescue her. The family finishes the session with a sense of direction; the therapist finishes it with the sense that he has been genuinely helpful to people he likes.

Joining is not a technique that can really be separated from changing a family; the therapist's joining changes things. Nor is it a process confined to one part of therapy. Joining is an operation which functions in counterpoint to every therapeutic intervention. The therapist joins and joins again many times during a session and during the course of therapy.

The deliberation of joining decreases, however, as therapy continues. Early in therapy, the therapist and family must concentrate on accommodating to each other and to the therapist's role as the leader. But as time goes on, these accommodations become more automatic. The therapist no longer has to think about joining. He can trust the patterns of the therapeutic system to alert him if the accommodations within the system need attention.

Employing joining techniques, as with other therapeutic techniques, can make a therapist feel like the centipede who was immobilized by having to decide which leg to move. But the therapist's effectiveness depends on his capacity to join while challenging. Expanding his repertory will ultimately make him a better therapist. And once he has become an expert reader of family feedback, the therapist will again be able to be spontaneous, confident that his behavior falls within the therapeutic system's accepted range.

4 Planning

If you flew over a flock of penguins, you might imagine that this was a convention of butlers—so precise a patterning of black and white and such stateliness of movement could belong to no other group. But as soon as you could get a real look at your subject, that hypothesis would be discarded. Butlers have arms, not flippers; they are human, and these creatures clearly are not. But what are they? As you saw one dive into the water to swim effortlessly away, you might decide that penguins were fish. Only closer acquaintance would lead you to discard this second hypothesis, and move toward the correct solution.

It is always a mistake, Sherlock Holmes warned, to theorize ahead of one's data. Planning treatment is an activity that can be engaged in only with an awareness of its limitations, as the fable of the penguin cautions. Family therapists learn, in effect, to theorize ahead of their data about a family, but always with awareness that a family's structure is never immediately available to a therapist. Only in the process of joining a family, probing its interactions and experiencing its governing structure, can a therapist get to know the transactions of that family. Any initial hypotheses will have to be tested in joining, and they may all be quickly discarded.

Nevertheless, an initial hypothesis can be invaluable to a therapist. Families come with different shapes and structures, and since form will affect function, families will respond to stresses in certain ways that are necessitated by their shape. Their shape will indicate possible functional areas and possible weak links in their structural arrangement.

The therapist forms an idea of the family as a whole upon first examination of certain basic aspects of its structure. From the simplest information gathered on a phone call setting up the first appointment, or recorded on a clinic intake sheet, the therapist can develop some assumptions about the family. For instance, how many people are in the family and where do they live? What are the ages of the family members? Is one of the normal transitional points that stress every family a factor here? The presenting problem may be another clue that suggests areas of possible strength and weakness in each client family. From these simple elements, the therapist will develop some hunches about the family to guide her first probes into the family organization.

The most immediate clue is family composition. Certain combinations indicate certain areas for exploration. The most commonly encountered family shapes are the pas de deux, three generation, shoe, accordion, fluctuating, and foster.

PAS DE DEUX FAMILIES

Suppose that a family consists of only two people. The therapist can guess that these two people probably rely on each other a great deal. If they are mother and child, the child may spend much time in the company of adults. She may have advanced verbal skills, and because of a high percentage of interaction with adults, she may become interested in adult issues before her peers and appear more mature. She may spend less time with peers than the usual child, having less in common with them, and she may be at a disadvantage in physical play. The mother is free, if she chooses, to give the child more individual attention than would be possible if there were a husband or other children to be concerned with. As a result, she may be very good at reading the child's moods, satisfying her needs, and answering her questions. She may, indeed, have a tendency to over-read the child, as she has no one else on whom to concentrate. She may have no one with whom to check her observations. The result can be an intense style of relating which fosters mutual dependence and mutual resentment at the same time.

Another example of the pas de deux family is the older couple whose children have left home. They are sometimes said to suffer from the empty nest syndrome. Still another example is the parent and adult single child who have lived together all the child's life.

Every family structure, no matter how viable in some cases, has areas of possible difficulty, or weak links in the chain. The two-person structure has the possibility of a lichen-like formation, in which the individuals become almost symbiotically dependent on each other. This is a possibility that the therapist will probe. If her observations indicate that overinvolvement is curtailing each member's potential functioning, the therapist will plan interventions to delineate the boundary between the dyad members while opening out the boundaries that keep each individual closed off from other relationships. The therapist may explore the family's extrafamilial sources of support or interest in order to challenge the "we are an island" view of the family reality.

THREE-GENERATION FAMILIES

The extended family with the various generations living close together is probably the most typical family shape, worldwide. Many therapists have emphasized the importance of working with three generations, regardless of possible geographic distancing. In the Western urban context, however, the multigeneration family tends to be more typical of lower middle class and low socioeconomic groups. Therefore, the therapist may tend to look at this family shape in terms of its deficits, instead of searching out the form's sources of adaptational strength.

The extended family shape contains within its multiple generations the possibility of specialization of function. The organization of support and cooperation in family tasks can be managed with an inherent flexibility, and often a true expertise. This type of organization requires a context in which the family and extrafamilial are continuous and harmonious. Like any family shape, the extended family needs a societal context that complements its operations.

In working with three-generation families, family therapists should guard against their penchant for separation. Therapists tend to want to delineate the boundaries of the nuclear family. In a family with a mother, grandmother, and a child, the family therapist's first question is often, "Who is parenting the child?" If the parenting functions are relegated to the grandmother, the map-maker inside of the therapist begins to devise strategies to reorganize the family shape so that the "real mother" takes over the major responsibility for parenting the child and the grandmother moves into the background. This adherence of the family therapist to the cultural norms should be shaken up a bit, since it may be that what is therapeutic for that three-generation family is to work within the cooperative system toward a differentiation of functions rather than to push for a structure that corresponds to the cultural norm.

It is important for the therapist to find out what is the idiosyncratic arrangement for this particular family. It may be that the grandmother is living with the daughter and grandchild. But it is also possible that the grandmother is the head of the house and that the mother and child function under her care. Is there a clearly delineated structure, with both adults living as equals and one acting as the child's primary parent? Are the adults cooperating in an organization with differentiated functions and expertise, or are the two adults struggling for positions of primacy? And in this last situation, is the child in coalition with one woman against the other?

There are many forms of three-generation families, ranging from the single parent, grandparent, and child combination, to the complex network of entire kin systems who need not live in the same house to wield great influence. It may be necessary for the therapist to find out who "the family" really is, how many members it has, and what is their level of contact with the extended network. The influence of the extended family on nuclear family functions should never be underrated.[1]

A possible weak link in the multigeneration family is the hierarchical organization. When an extended three-generation family comes to therapy with one of its members as the symptom bearer, the therapist will explore cross-generational coalitions that may be scapegoating one family member or rendering certain holons dysfunctional.

In some disorganized extended families, adults may function in a disengaged, centrifugal way. In such cases, executive functions, including child rearing, may remain underdefined and "fall between the cracks." This problem is often seen in poor, overburdened families living in slums without societal systems of support. Clarifying boundaries among holons can help differentiate functions and facilitate cooperation.[2]

SHOE FAMILIES

The large family is not as common as it once was in this culture. At one time, having many children was the norm. Children were considered a family asset. Times have changed, but the structural relationship found in most large families has not. Whenever institutions become large, authority must be delegated. With many children in a household, usually one and perhaps several of the older children are given parental responsibilities. These parental children take over child-rearing functions as the representatives of the parents.

This arrangement works well as long as the parental child's responsibilities are clearly defined by the parents and fall within the capabilities of the child, given her level of maturity. The parental child is put in a position in which she is excluded from the sibling subsystem and kicked upward to the parental subsystem. This position has some attractive features, since the child has direct access to the parents, and it can increase the child's executive skills. The relationship has worked well for millennia. Many therapists are former parental children. But the structure of a large family can break down at this point, and a therapist must be aware of this possibility.

The potential exists that parental children will become symptomatic when they are given responsibilities that they cannot handle, or are not given the authority to carry out their responsibilities. Parental children are, by definition, caught in the middle. The parental child feels excluded from the sibling context and not truly accepted by the parental holon. The important socialization context of the sibling subsystem is handicapped. Furthermore, the nurturance functions that the younger children need from the parents may be blocked by the parental child.

In therapy, it can be useful to employ boundary-making techniques that reorganize the parental subsystem without the parental child, and to conduct sessions among the siblings alone in which the position of the parental child in the sibling subsystem becomes reorganized. Or if the parental subsystem is already overloaded, the responsibility for supporting the parental subsystem may be distributed more fairly among the other siblings.

ACCORDION FAMILIES

In some families one parent is away for long periods of time. Military families are the classical example. When one spouse leaves, the spouse who stays must take on additional nurturant, executive, and guiding functions or the children will go without. The parental functions are concentrated into one person for part of each cycle. Families may crystallize in the shape of a one-parent family. The spouse at home assumes additional functions at the expense of spouse collaboration. The children may function to further the separation of the parents, even to crystallize them in the roles of "good father and bad, deserting mother" in an organization that tends to evict the peripheral parent.

Accordion families may come to therapy if the job of the traveling parent changes and she becomes a permanent figure in the family organization. At this point, there needs to be a shift in the way in which the family organizes its functions, for the old program handicaps the evolution of new functions that include the absent spouse. The peripheral parent must be reincluded in a meaningful position.

In these situations, as in other transitional situations, therapy will include not only restructuring maneuvers but also educational ones. The family must come to understand that, in effect, they are a "new" family. This concept is a rather difficult one to accept, since the "parts" of the family have been together for a long time; only the shape of the family is new.

FLUCTUATING FAMILIES

Some families move constantly from one place to another, like the ghetto family who leave when the rent is too long overdue, or the corporation executive who is transferred again and again by the parent company. In other families, it is the family composition that fluctuates. This occurs most frequently when a single parent has serial love affairs. A father may pass from girl friend to girl friend, each one a potential spouse and parent. This configuration may not be apparent to the therapist on initial contact, but it will become clear as she works with the family over time.

If the shifting context involves significant adults, it is important for the therapist to get a history, to determine if what seems to be a stable organization is in effect transitional. Part of the therapist's function will then be to help the family define its organizational structure clearly. If the shifting context involves location, there is a loss of systems of support, both family and community. The family is bereft. Children who have lost their peer network and must enter a new school context may find themselves dysfunctional. If the family becomes the only context of support in a shifting world, its ability to contact the extrafamilial may suffer.

The therapist must realize that when the family loses its context by relocation, its members will enter into crisis and tend to function at a lower level of competence than in circumstances where the extrafamilial context is supportive. Therefore, assessment of the level of competence both of the family as an organism and of the individual members becomes a relevant issue. It is essential not to assume that the crisis is a product of pathology in the family. The family holon is always a part of a larger context. With the larger context in disruption, the family will evidence disruption.

FOSTER FAMILIES

A foster child is by definition a temporary family member. Agency workers make it clear that the foster family is not to become attached to the child; a parent-child relationship is to be avoided. Nevertheless, parent-child bonds often do become established, only to be broken when the child moves to a new foster home or back to her family of origin.

A potential problem with this family shape is that sometimes the family organizes like a nonfoster family. The child is incorporated into the family system. If she then develops symptoms, they may be the result of stresses within the family organism. But the therapist and family may assume that the child's symptoms are the product of her experiences prior to her entrance into this family, or that they are the product of internalized pathology, since she is a foster child and technically not a family member.

The relationship of the symptom to the family organization should be assessed. If the symptomatology is the product of the child's entrance into a new system, then the system is functioning as if in a transitional crisis. On the contrary, if the child is already fully integrated into the family, her symptoms are family organized and related to the stresses that other family members express in other ways.

In the latter situation, an additional complexity of the foster family shape is the presence of the agency. Foster family agencies, which invest a lot of time and effort in developing good foster parents, tend to be very protective of them. They may operate in a way that hinders the possibility of accommodation between the child and the host family. In these cases the therapist must consider bringing the agency worker into the therapeutic context and working with the agency worker as a cotherapist to help the total family organism, including the child.

Intake information often tells something not only about these kinds of family composition, but also about the family's developmental stage. Family development implies transitions. Families change in adapting to different circumstances. Occurrences in the family's developmental stage may therefore be threatening the family equilibrium. Many families come to therapy precisely because they are in a transitional period, in which demands for change and the counterdeviation mechanisms activated by those demands are handicapping family function. These problems of discontinuity are found in stepparent families and families with a ghost.

STEPPARENT FAMILIES

When a stepparent is added to a family unit, she must go through a process of integration, which will prove to be more or less successful. She may make less than a full commitment to the new family, or the original unit may keep her peripheral. The children may increase their demands on their natural parent, exacerbating his problem with divided loyalties. In cases where the children lived away from their natural parent until his remarriage, they must now accommodate to both their own parent and their stepparent.

Crises in this family shape are comparable to problems in a new family organism; they should be seen as normal. Western culture postulates instant family formation. After the ritual, whether legal or paralegal, the members of a "blended" family rush into family holons. But time has not yet given them functional legitimacy. A therapist may have to help the family by introducing designs for gradual evolution. In some cases, it may be useful in the beginning for the members of the two original families to maintain their functional boundaries, meeting as two cooperating halves to resolve issues as the family moves toward a one-organism shape.

FAMILIES WITH A GHOST

A family which has experienced death or desertion may have problems reassigning the tasks of the missing member. Sometimes a family will establish the attitude that if the mother had lived, she would have known what to do. Taking over the mother's functions becomes an act of disloyalty to her memory. Old coalitions may be respected, as if the mother were still alive.

Problems in these families may be experienced by family members as issues of incomplete mourning. But if the therapist operates on this assumption, she may crystallize the family instead of helping them move toward a new organization. From the therapeutic point of view, this is a family in transition. Previous shapes are handicapping the development of new structures.

As the therapist thinks over all of the initial information on a family, a speculative family structure takes shape. It acknowledges the configuration that the family reports as basic. It includes elements of the family's developmental stage and the possible problems inherent in that stage. If the family's religion, economic status, or ethnic background are known, this information is included. Finally, the picture incorporates the presenting problem. If an infant is failing to thrive, the therapist will probe for dysfunction in the mother-child interactions. If a child "won't mind," the therapist will probe for an alliance within the family hierarchy that is giving the child adult support for disobedience.

Certain symptoms are a clear indication of certain family structural arrangements. Therefore, the "presenting problem" triggers any trained therapist's imagination. It immediately evokes the page of some book of psychology, the face of some child seen previously, or the shape of another family with similar problems. These images are useful in forming the initial set of hypotheses with which the therapist will approach the family.

OUT-OF-CONTROL FAMILIES

In families where one of the members presents symptoms related to control, the therapist assumes that there are problems in one or all of certain areas: the hierarchical organization of the family, the implementation of executive functions in the parental subsystem, and the proximity of family members.

Issues of control vary, depending on the developmental stage of family members. In families with young children, one of the most common problems to appear in a child guidance clinic is the preschooler described by the parents as a "monster" who will not obey any rules. When a fifty-pound tyrant terrorizes an entire family, it must be assumed that she has an accomplice. For a three-foot tyrant to be taller than the rest of the family members, she has to be standing on the shoulders of one of the adults. In all cases, the therapist may safely assume that the spouses disqualify each other, which leaves the triangulated tyrant in a position of power that is frightening to her as well as to the family.

The therapeutic goal in this situation is the reorganization of the family, with the parents cooperating and the child appropriately demoted. The development of a clear hierarchy, in which the parents have control of the executive subsystem, requires a therapeutic input that affects the entire parental holon.

In families with adolescents, the issues of control may be related to the inability of the parents to move from the stage of concerned parents of young children to respectful parents of young adolescents. In this situation, old programs that served well for the family when the children were young interfere in the development of a new family shape. The children may feel more comfortable with changes in their development, whereas the parents have not yet evolved new alternatives for their own stage in life.

An adolescent child may also be so overinvolved with a hovering parent that no action of the child remains unnoticed. In these situations, blocking the overinvolved transaction may increase the encounters between the parental holon and the child, which may help in the exploration of alternatives.

In general, the best route for the therapist when dealing with families of adolescents in conflict is to travel the middle of the road. She will support the parents' rights to make certain demands and request respect for their position. She will also support the adolescents' demands for change.

In families with delinquent children, the parents' control is dependent on their presence. Rules exist only as long as the parents are there to implement them. The child learns that in one context there are certain rules, but these rules do not operate in others. In this organization, the parents tend to make a high number of controlling responses, which are often ineffective. The parent makes a controlling demand, the child does not obey, the parent makes another demand, and so on. There is a mutual agreement that after a certain number of parental demands, the child will respond.

Communication patterns tend to be chaotic in these families. People do not expect to be heard, and relationship messages are more important than the content. Communications seem to be organized around small, disconnected, affect-carrying bits or transactions.

When these families have several children, the sibling subsystem can be an important context for beginning to organize a new family shape and for creating meaningful boundaries. Other therapeutic techniques for these families have been described elsewhere by Minuchin and others.[3]

In families with child abuse, the system cannot control the parents' destructive responses to children. Usually the parents are devoid of supportive systems. They respond to the children as if they were only a continuation of themselves. Every action of the child is felt by the parent to be a personal response. Parents in this situation do not have their own adult context in which they are competent. The family becomes too much the only field in which the parent expresses power and competence, which emerge as aggression. Just as people hit each other only in clinches, only overinvolved subsystems tend to produce abusing parents.

Sometimes the child abuse family is organized around an overinvolved dyad, one parent and child. Usually this is the mother and child, with the father attacking them indiscriminately, as an enemy alliance. In these families, abuse between the parents is overflowing to the child.

The family of the infant who fails to thrive is sometimes put in the same category as the abused child family, because the effect in both cases is to endanger the child. However, the characteristics of the family are different. Failure to thrive involves not a situation of proximity but, on the contrary, an inability of the parents to respond to the child's needs. In effect, this is a disengaged organization. The mother is not feeding the child as much as she needs. She is being distracted when the child is at the breast or bottle. In these situations therapeutic techniques involve engaging the parents, instead of the boundary making techniques that are indicated in child abuse situations.

There are two types of families in which children have school phobias. In one, the school phobia is a manifestation of a delinquentlike organization. In the other group, the situation is similar to families who have psychosomatic children. There is an overinvolvement between the child and some family member which hooks the child into remaining at home as a companion.

PSYCHOSOMATIC FAMILIES

When the presenting complaint is a psychosomatic problem in one of the family members, the structure of the family is one that includes an overemphasis on nurturing roles. The family seems to function best when someone is sick. The characteristics of such families include overprotection, enmeshment, or overinvolvement of family members with each other, an inability to resolve conflicts, a tremendous concern for the maintenance of peace or avoidance of conflict, and an extreme rigidity. This is not the rigidity of the challenge, but rather the rigidity of water, which lets itself be grasped only to return to its original form. These families look like the normal, all-American family. They are benign neighbors. They do not fight. They are very loyal and very protective— the ideal family.

One of the problems that these families present to the therapist is that they are so likeable. They seem eager to respond. The therapist may feel that they are cooperating with her, only to find herself frustrated again and again by the problems of these families, as well as by her easy induction into the molasses of their attitude of peace at any price.

READING STRUCTURE FROM EARLY TRANSACTIONS

The skeletal information that can be gathered from an intake sheet or a phone conversation evokes the possibility of certain family shapes and problem areas. This cognitive schema is useful in helping the therapist organize her initial contact with the family. But only in the formation of the therapeutic system can the information to buttress, clarify, or refute the initial hypothesis be gathered. The cases that follow demonstrate how to read structure from early transactions.

In the Malcolm family the identified patient is Michael, age 23. While away at college, Michael had a psychotic break during his senior year. He and his wife of four months came back to the city, where Michael was hospitalized. Coming to the initial session are Michael and his wife Cathi, Michael's parents, and his younger brother Doug, who is a college freshman.

Reading this information on the intake sheet, the therapist notes that during one year this family has experienced the marriage of one child and the loss of the other to college. Questions immediately come to mind. Is this a family that has difficulty separating? Has the vacuum created by the absence of the younger brother caused instability in Michael's family? If Michael has had difficulties separating from his parents, have these exacerbated the problems of forming his own marriage relationship?

As the Malcolm family enters the room, Mr. and Mrs. Malcolm sit on one side of the room. Michael's wife sits down opposite them. Michael walks in and, looking at no one in particular, says, "Where shall I sit?" His mother folds her arms, then extends a hand, pointing to a chair. "I guess you sit next to your wife," she says. Michael responds, "I think I'll sit next to my wife."

Michael's question was not directed to one person. The fact that his mother answered suggests that there is a great deal of proximity between Michael and his mother. If the position of the two spouse units were more clearly defined, Michael might have directed the question to his wife, or his wife might have answered. More likely, Michael would not have asked the question in the first place; he would automatically have sat next to his wife. The wording of the mother's reply also suggests a closeness with her son, or at least an ambivalence about Michael's marriage.

Much more information is needed, to verify this speculation. The therapist cannot decide on a definition of the family structure and problems until he has seen many more such transactions. Furthermore, there are other relationships he must find out about. What is the relationship of the mother and father? If this mother is overly close to her son, perhaps there is distance, or even conflict, in her relationship with her husband. What is the position of the younger son? Was he a stabilizer in the family until he left for college, and did his absence generate an instability which contributed to Michael's breakdown? Or did Michael, in spite of absence and marriage, remain closely involved in his parents' transactions, leaving Doug in a more distant position? How successful have Michael and Cathi been in forming a marriage (according to the intake sheet, their relationship already has "problems")? What about Cathi's side of the family?

Nevertheless, the therapist already has a structural hypothesis to guide his first probes. His hunch is that the mother and Michael form an overinvolved dyad which keeps the father and Cathi peripheral.

This kind of hunch gives the therapist a working blueprint. In the course of therapy the blueprint will be expanded, modified, or perhaps scrapped altogether. But the therapist has a framework for his early contacts with the family. He will probe the hypothesized closeness of Michael to his mother. The relationships of Michael and Cathi, and of Mr. and Mrs. Malcolm, will be analyzed. If the hypothesis is borne out by further data, the therapist will work to strengthen both spouse subsystems, not only by working to delineate the boundary between them, but also by helping to increase the rewards of participation in the individual subsystems. The structural hypothesis from the intake sheet data, apparently supported by the early therapeutic contact, has given the therapist a working idea of where he is, and even where he may be going.

In the Jackson family, four children, aged 14, 17, 19, and 20, are living at home with their mother. The intake sheet notes that five older children have left home, though one of the older daughters and her infant are living with the Jacksons until the daughter can find a job. The identified patient is Joanne, age 17. She has been referred by the school for low grades and difficulty getting along with peers.

From this intake information, the therapist notes that the family is in the stage when the children separate. All of the children remaining at home are adolescents, presumably involved in building their own lives independent of the family—a process already begun some years before by the older children. The therapist hypothesizes that Joanne is having difficulty separating.

The family enters the room with a great deal of joking and kidding. One of the sons is carrying a radio tuned loud. Everyone talks at once. The mother, who seems older than her 48 years, sits in the corner, saying very little. Joanne appears to function as the family's executive head, giving her siblings various orders and seeing that they are followed. Looking at the 14-year-old-boy, the therapist says, "What's your name?" The child is silent. Joanne looks at her brother and says, "Answer the man." He does. Another child asks to go to the bathroom. The therapist says, "Sure, go ahead." "Don't forget to come back," Joanne warns him. Later, the therapist asks what the grandson's name is. Joanne rises and picks up the child. "This is Tyrone," she replies.

From these transactions, it is clear that the therapist's intake sheet hypothesis must be radically expanded. It now appears that Joanne functions as the head of a large, disorganized family, taking over from a depressed parent. The therapist hypothesizes that Joanne's numerous duties at home, as parental child in a disorganized family, are interfering with her age-appropriate activities, such as attending school.

If this hypothesis is correct, the therapist knows what the treatment plan must be. Joanne has to be relieved of some of the burdens of the parental child. The therapist must work with the mother to help her resolve some of her difficulties and become more forceful in organizing the family. Some of the executive functioning must be divided among the other children. Probably all the children living at home will need help with the process of separation.

From a systems point of view, the concept of family shape in these cases has limited usefulness. The therapist must never forget that in actually gathering data, she is inside the system she is studying. Furthermore, the family is never a static entity. Formulating the family shape from initial data is a useful first step, but it is only a first step. The therapist must move beyond it almost immediately, to the actual dance of therapy.

5 Change

All family therapists agree on the need to challenge the dysfunctional aspects of family homeostasis. The degree to which the challenge should be taken is a moot point, however, and the methods and targets of the challenge vary depending on the therapist's theoretical worldview. Technique is the pathway to change, but it is the therapist's conceptualization of the family dynamics and the process of change that gives the way its direction. The effectiveness of a particular technique cannot be evaluated without an understanding of the therapist's goal. The way in which theory prescribes therapeutic techniques is illustrated by three positions in family therapy—the existential framework as represented by Carl Whitaker, the strategic school as represented by Jay Haley and Chloe Madanes, and the structural position.[1]

Whitaker sees the family as a system in which each member is equally significant. Each member must be individually changed to change the whole. Consequently, he challenges each family member, undermining each person's comfortable allegiance to the family's way of apprehending life. Each individual is made to experience the absurdity of accepting the family's idiosyncratic worldview as valid.

Whitaker's sessions seem undirected, because he accepts and tracks any family member's communication. He rarely challenges the content of a communication, but he does not accept it either. Any statement presented as complete is turned into a fragment; like James Joyce, Whitaker creates a revolution in the grammar of life. He brings up an association with his own life, an anecdote about his brother, a slightly different comment another family member made, or a joke: "What would he do if God retired?" Though seemingly random, his interventions all are directed to challenging the meaning that people give to events.

Whitaker's assumption seems to be that out of his challenge to form, creative processes in individual members as well as in the family as a whole can arise. Out of this experiential soup, a better arrangement among family members can result.

Whitaker is a destroyer of crystallized forms. If a family member enters a dialog, it is not long before Whitaker asks a third person a question that is related to the theme tangentially, if at all. The content of family members' communications is stretched to touch areas that are human universals, but which people own uneasily: rage, killing, seducing, paranoid fears, incest. All of it is presented casually, amid commonplace statements.

Whitaker will comment himself on an issue, relating a communication to another person, fantasy, or memory. He also links family members again and again, while at the same time destroying their connections, like a sculptor carving a wax statue with tools that are white hot.

Whitaker's therapy is dazzling by the range of his interventions. He uses humor, indirection, seduction, indignation, primary process, boredom, and even falling asleep as equally powerful instruments of contact and challenge. By the end of therapy every family member has been touched by Whitaker's distorting magic. Each member feels challenged, misunderstood, accepted, rejected, or insulted. But he has been put in contact with a less familiar part of himself.

Whitaker's techniques make sense only within his theoretical schema. In this existential formulation, the therapist is not responsible for monitoring the development of new structures, and it is not his responsibility if these do not appear.

The strategic formulation represented by Haley and Madanes differs markedly. Their techniques are goal oriented—directed toward alleviation of specific dysfunctional aspects of the family. It is very much the therapist's responsibility to monitor development and produce improvement.

The strategic school sees the family as a complex system, differentiated into hierarchically arranged subsystems. A dysfunction in one subsystem can be expressed analogically in another; in particular, the organization of family members around the symptom is taken to be an analogical statement of dysfunctional structures. By rearranging the organization around the symptom, the therapist can release isomorphic changes in the entire system.

In this strategic formulation, the identified patient is seen as carrying the symptom to protect the family. At the same time, the symptom is maintained by a family organization in which the family members occupy incongruous hierarchies. For instance, the identified patient is in an inferior position in relation to the family members who take care of him, but he is in a superior position by not improving under their care. The therapeutic techniques are directed to challenging the heart of the dysfunctional structure: the organization of the symptom.

The strategic school has made the supervisory holon the focus of their exploration in therapy. In their work with severely disturbed young adults, the cornerstone of their techniques is the redistribution of clearly allocated power in the family. By organizing family holons so that each one has a defined hierarchy, and by putting the heads of the executive holons in control, they create a field in which autonomy, responsibility, and cooperation are played out.

To challenge the restrictive ways in which crystallized family systems prescribe a view of reality to the family members, Haley and Madanes suggest that the patients pretend that the world is different. A depressed husband is to pretend he feels depressed. His wife is to judge whether he is pretending. The control that the husband has kept over the wife, by not improving while remaining in a powerless position, is changed to a game in which the spouses play different power arrangements.

In a case in which a child develops symptoms of being afraid, a fearful mother becomes competent, protecting the child from his symptom, while in effect the child is protecting the mother from hers. The therapist asks the mother to pretend to be afraid of robbers. The child pretends to protect her. Now the problem of protection is transformed. The hierarchy of mother and child is realigned by the pretend technique, for a child protects his mother only in play.

These cases demonstrate how the techniques of the strategic school are governed by the theoretical schema. These therapists use many different techniques in different family situations. But the governing concept is the specific goal for family change.

Whitaker's approach is difficult to use unless the therapist has the same theoretical view and skills. The strategic school techniques, how-

ever, are described with such specificity and their intention seems so
clear that they appeal to the therapist interested in craft. It is therefore
important to understand that, without the strategic conceptualization of
the meaning of dysfunction and change, these techniques lose their effectiveness and become just unrelated tools.

The structural approach sees the family as an organism: a complex
system that is underfunctioning. The therapist undermines the existing
homeostasis, creating crises that jar the system toward the development
of a better functioning organization. Thus, the structural approach has
elements of both the existential and the strategic frameworks. Like the
strategist, the structuralist realigns significant organizations to produce
change in the entire system. And like the existentialist, the structuralist
challenges the family's accepted reality with an orientation toward
growth. Structural family therapy partakes of the existentialist's concern for growth and the strategist's concern for cure.

The techniques of structural therapy lead to family reorganization by
challenging the family organization. The word *challenge* highlights the
nature of the dialectic struggle between family and therapist within the
therapeutic system. The word does not imply harsh maneuvers, or confrontation, though at times both may be indicated. It suggests a search
for new patterns, as well as the fact that, as in the work of Siva, goddess
of destruction, the old order must be undermined, to allow for the formation of the new.

There are three main strategies of structural family therapy, each of
which is served by a group of techniques. The three strategies are challenging the symptom, challenging the family structure, and challenging
the family reality.

CHALLENGING THE SYMPTOM

Families coming to therapy after a prolonged struggle have usually
identified one family member as the problem. They pour out to the
therapist their struggle, the solutions they have tried, and the failure of
every attempt. The therapist, however, enters the therapeutic situation
with the assumption that the family is wrong. The problem is not the
identified patient, but certain family interactional patterns. The solutions the family has tried are stereotyped repetitions of ineffective transactions, which can only generate heightened affect without producing
change. By observing the family members' organization around the
symptom and the symptom bearer, the therapist may gain a "transac-

tional biopsy" of the preferential responses of the family organism—the responses that the family is still using inappropriately to meet the current situation.

The strategic therapist sees the symptom as a protective solution: the symptom bearer sacrifices himself to defend the family homeostasis. The structuralist, regarding the family as an organism, sees this protection not as a purposeful, "helpful" response, but as a reaction of an organism under stress. The other family members are equally symptomatic. The therapist's task, then, is to challenge the family's definition of the problem and the nature of their response. Challenge can be direct or indirect, explicit or implicit, straightforward or paradoxical. The goal is to change or reframe the family's view of the problem, pushing its members to search for alternative behavioral, cognitive, and affective responses. The techniques involved in these strategies are enactment, focusing, and achieving intensity.

The Mitchells, a family of professional parents with a 12-year-old girl and a five-year-old boy, came to therapy because the boy urinates on the floor whenever he is angry at his mother. The parents had tried a variety of approaches to no avail, including rewards, such as involving the child in pleasurable activities, and punishments, such as withholding affection and spanking. Both parents and child feel hopelessly depleted, helpless, and guilty. They are tremendously overinvolved with each other around the symptom.

In an initial interview held at the therapist's home, the therapist uses his dog as a cotherapist: an expert in defining turf by urinating. He invites the child to follow the dog around the garden and observe its techniques. He further detoxifies the symptom by suggesting more destructive channels for anger than the one the boy is using: has he ever thought of standing on his sister's bed and peeing in her face? Humor helps the parents regain their perspective. Now they can see the child as a relatively small five-year-old whose contacting responses are incompetent.

The therapist then explores alternative ways of expressing resentment and disagreement in this family. He examines the different intensities of each parent's involvement with the symptom, the meaning the symptom holds for each family member, and the utilization of the symptom in the spouse and sibling subsystems. The symptom is redefined as a way of reengaging the mother, who has recently changed her relationship with the child and her husband. This redefinition opens up new perspectives on the conflictual relationship between the spouses, the distancing between the father and son, and the privileged position of the son in the sibling subsystem. As the family members find themselves exploring new territory, their mood changes, becoming more intense and at the same time more hopeful.

CHALLENGING THE FAMILY STRUCTURE

The worldview of family members depends to a great extent on their positions in different family holons. If there is overinvolvement, the members' freedom to function is restricted by the rules of the holon. If there is underinvolvement, the members may be isolated, and lack support. Increasing or decreasing the proximity between the members of significant holons may bring forth alternative ways of thinking, feeling, and acting that have been inhibited by subsystem participation.

When the therapist joins the family, he becomes a participant in the system that he is attempting to transform. As he experiences the family's transactions, he begins to form an experiential diagnosis of the family functioning. This family map indicates the position of family members vis-à-vis one another. It reveals coalitions, affiliations, explicit and implicit conflicts, and the ways family members group themselves in conflict resolution. It identifies family members who operate as detourers of conflict and family members who function as switchboards. The map charts the nurturers, healers, and scapegoaters. Its delineation of the boundaries between subsystems indicates what movement there is and suggests possible areas of strength or dysfunction.

Areas of dysfunction in a family frequently involve either overaffiliation or underaffiliation. In great measure, therefore, therapy is a process of monitoring proximity and distance. The therapist, though constrained by the system's demands, is also an outsider. He can shift position and work in alternative subsystems, challenging the family members' own delineation of their roles and functions. The techniques involved in this strategy are boundary making, unbalancing, and teaching complementarity.

The Dexter family, for example, composed of two parents in their thirties and two boys, Mark, age nine, and Ronny, age four, came into therapy because Ronny has serious eczema which is exacerbated by his constant, uncontrollable scratching. Mrs. Dexter is overinvolved with Ronny. Whenever she pays attention to Mark, Ronny begins to scratch, irritating his eczema and reinvolving his mother with himself. The father, a competent teacher, has the capacity for involvement with his children, but his wife's overinvolvement with Ronny leaves him in a peripheral relationship with his younger son. He thinks that his wife is too involved with Ronny. Both parents, though overprotective, are concerned, child-centered people. The relationship between the spouses is somewhat distant.

The family therapist watches Ronny's constant engagement of his mother for a few minutes, experiencing the enmeshment of this dyad and the boundaries around the dyad that exclude the father and Mark. Then he organizes a task. He instructs the parents to talk without letting Ronny intrude. Whenever Mrs. Dexter looks at Ronny, Mr. Dexter is to re-engage her attention.

This boundary delineation produces Ronny's usual response. He begins to whimper, then cry, jumping up and down in his chair and scratching furiously. But with the therapist's help the parents ignore him, continuing to talk to each other. Mark, obviously the parental child, tosses a toy to Ronny, engaging him in a playful, slightly aggressive transaction. Soon Ronny throws the toy at Mark and runs to his mother. Mr. Dexter attracts his wife's attention again.

At first Ronny returns to his mother every minute or so. But as she does not respond, he begins to function differently. He explores the room, then picks up a large toy and begins to toss it to Mark. His motor activity becomes less hesitant, and his scratching ceases completely. At the same time, as Mrs. Dexter's almost ticlike hovering over Ronny disappears, she becomes more direct in her contact with her husband. He makes some criticism, and instead of detouring by engaging with Ronny, she responds by confronting her husband directly.

It seems that certain behaviors are signaled in the overinvolved dyad of the mother and Ronny. The disappearance of this signaling because of the therapist's boundary delineation allows the boy's usually underutilized skills to appear.

In this situation, the therapist's intervention has changed the family members' contexts. An overinvolved pair has been slightly distanced. As a result, Ronny moves into participation with his older brother, forming a dyad that requires him to function more competently. The mother moves from a situation in which she is exclusively a parent, nurturing and controlling, to a conflict negotiation with a peer in the spouse holon. The changes in subsystem participation have produced a change in functioning, which enables coping capacities to appear.

By challenging the rules that constrain people's experience, the therapist actualizes submerged aspects of their repertory. As a result, the family members perceive themselves and one another as functioning in a different way. The modification of context produces a change in experience.

Another technique for changing the nature of involvement is to focus the family members' experience on the reality of being a holon. The therapist attempts to change the family members' epistemology, moving them from a definition of the self as a separate entity to a definition of the self as part of a whole.

An individual therapist tells the patient, "Change yourself, work with yourself, so you will grow." The family therapist makes a statement of a different order. Family members can change only if there is a change in the contexts within which they live. The family therapist's message is, therefore, "Help the other person change, which will change yourself as you relate to him and will change both of you within the holon."

CHALLENGING THE FAMILY REALITY

Patients come to therapy because reality, as they have constructed it, is unworkable. All types of therapy therefore, depend on a challenge to their constructs. Psychodynamic therapy postulates that the patient's conscious reality is too narrow; there is an unconscious world that he must explore. Behavioral therapy suggests that the patient has mis-learned aspects of how to deal with his contexts. Family therapy postulates that transactional patterns depend on and contain the way people experience reality. Therefore, to change the way family members look at reality requires the development of new ways of interacting in the family. The techniques used in this strategy are cognitive constructs, paradoxical interventions, and emphasizing strength.

The therapist takes the data that the family offers and reorganizes it. The conflictual and stereotyped reality of the family is given a new framing. As the family members experience themselves and one another differently, new possibilities appear.

For example, the Gilbert family, composed of a mother and father in their forties and their daughter Judy, aged 15, came to therapy because Judy has anorexia nervosa.[2] The family presentation of the problem is that they are a typical, normal family, with a daughter who was perfect before the illness transformed her. For the past year they have been try-ing to help their daughter, changing their relationship to her on the ad-vice of friends, minister, pediatrician, and child psychiatrist. By now they feel helpless and considerably frightened.

The therapist meets with the family at lunch and they all eat together. The therapist asks the parents to help their daughter survive by making her eat. The daughter refuses to eat and responds to her parents with a broad range of surprisingly sophisticated insults. The therapist focuses on these insults, pointing out that the daughter is strong enough to defeat both parents. His intervention produces a reframing. The parents, who are overinvolved with the daughter and accustomed to triangulating her in their unresolved conflicts, close ranks. Feeling attacked and defeated, they simultaneously increase their distance from the daughter, removing their overprotection and overcontrol. The parents and therapist together demand that the daughter, who is suddenly perceived as strong, competent, and stubborn, monitor her own body.

This type of reconstruction can elicit a startled new look at reality, in which the potential for change is suddenly perceived.

6 Reframing

Humans are storytellers, myth-makers, framers of realities. Our ancestors drew the relevant reality of their time in the caves of Altamira, and peoples have shared their beliefs of what is significant reality in oral tradition, religious myth, history, and poetry. Anthropologists unearth the structural arrangement of societies by searching for the deeper meaning of myth.

In a playground in Central Park, a Puerto Rican mother watches her three-year-old playing in the sand box. An older woman tells her in Spanish that her son has a very nice *cuadro* (picture or image). She says that he will grow up to become a teacher. The prediction obviously pleases the mother, who smiles at the older woman while she brushes the sand from the child's knees.

A child's *cuadro* floats above his head, for everybody who is knowledgeable to see and transmit. Puerto Rican parents search for a child's *cuadro,* unaware that they are contributing to its construction. But every family, not only Puerto Rican, stamps upon its members the unique shape that identifies them as belonging to that family. This image, which individual psychologists see as role, is an ongoing interpersonal process. People are continuously molded by their contexts and the characteristics elicited by contexts.

Families, too, have a dynamic *cuadro* growing out of their own histories which frames their identities as social organisms. When they come to therapy, they bring this geography of their life as they define it. They have made their own assessment of their problems, their strengths, and their possibilities. They are asking the therapist to help with the reality that they have framed.

The therapist's first problem in joining the family is to define the therapeutic reality. Therapy is a goal-oriented enterprise, to which not all truths are relevant. By observing the family members' transactions in the therapeutic system, the therapist selects the data that will facilitate problem solving.

Therapy starts, therefore, with the clash between two framings of reality. The family's framing is relevant for the continuity and maintenance of the organism more or less as it is; the therapeutic framing is related to the goal of moving the family toward a more differentiated and competent dealing with their dysfunctional reality.

As an example of family myth-making, take the way the Minuchin family framed its reality when I was around eleven years old. I was supposed to be responsible, a day dreamer, and a child with ten thumbs. My sister was supposed to be socially competent, flighty, but efficient. My brother, eight years younger, came into a family in which labels had already been distributed, so we pegged on him the frames that were left— bright, easygoing, able, and irresponsible. The way in which the frames included and excluded experiences was quite simple: if my brother responded in a responsible way to family tasks, that behavior was framed as his being unusually able and intelligent; if I was not responsible, this was framed as unusually inefficient; and so it went. Our experiences were labeled in the "appropriate" way to fit our family truth. There were elaborations on these myths. I remember the "Balatin" family, whom my parents used to present as an example where the children were always competent. Not until my preadolescence did I realize that my parents were actually saying in Yiddish *ba-laten kinder,* or "other peoples' children," and I was alone in the construction of this mythical family; my brother and sister did not share this "shaming" family with me. It took many years of extrafamilial experience and the help of our respective spouses and children for us to modify, expand, and delete such frames.

We, the children, framed our parents in equally inflexible boxes. Our father was just, honest, and authoritarian, with a strict code of ethics that we could violate at our own peril; our mother was concerned, available, and protective, except that as our house was in just the right state of cleanliness and order, any breaking of this order was a transgression. We also had frames for both father-mother and sibling transactions. We were part of an extended patriarchal family, since our grandparents and the families of our paternal aunt, our maternal uncle, and a cousin all lived in contiguous houses. In this organism our family had a clearly delineated niche. My father was the responsible, fair arbiter of conflicts; my Aunt Esther and my mother shared the protective, fairy-godmother function for all their nieces and nephews.

Since our grandfather was a patriarch in the Jewish community that comprised about one-third of the total population of four thousand in our town, our family had a position in the clan that "demanded" fulfillment of that frame. We knew all the citizens of our town and had a relationship to them as buyers, sellers, neighbors, or friends, and we were participant members of the social life of the town. The combination in this ecological niche, which included my father's business, my horse, the school, and the chief of police whose mechanic son married the woman who had an hysterical pregnancy, framed my experiences and gave them meaning. All the parts of this framing had a different weight; the continuous transactions in my nuclear family gave intensity to certain definitions of "who-I-was-and-who-we-were" that my relationship with Tenerany, the son of the owner of the town newspaper, did not have. But my family was definitely a holon in a larger world, and our life was in context.

In my family there were problems, habitual problem solvers, and preferred solutions. When there were problems that my immediate family could not resolve, the aunts and uncles were there as helpers, as was my Aunt Sofia when my mother felt depressed after my grandmother's death, or my Uncle Elias when my father lost his business in the Depression.

When I was eleven years old, I needed to go to school away from home, since my home town had only five grades, and I lived for a year with the family of my Aunt Sofia. (Although my aunt was married for over fifty years to my Uncle Bernard, until his death, in my nuclear family the head-of-the-house position was always given to the member of my parents' family and not to the in-law). The year I spent in her house was the worst of my entire life. Away from home, friends, and familiar context, I grew depressed, had nightmares, felt isolated, was bullied in school by a bunch of "city kids," did poorly in my studies, and failed two subjects. I probably needed psychological help, only nobody noticed how I felt. The next year was somewhat better. I moved to the house of a cousin who had young children, shared a room with another cousin my age, and developed a friendship with three other adolescents. We formed a four-musketeers club that lasted throughout high school, so that by the time my family moved to the city, I had already developed a support system.

The point is that when I was quite dysfunctional at age eleven, if my family had decided I needed help, they would have gone the usual route of asking a cousin to tutor or talk to me, since solutions were usually found within the family. If there had been family therapists in Argentina at that time and we had come to one, I am sure the scenario they presented would have been along the lines of "solutions" that were already familiar at home: my father would have insisted on the need for more responsible work, my mother would have increased her concern and nurturance, and my younger sister and my aunt would have joined my mother in expressing concern about me. In the end, they all would have explicitly followed my father's lead, since he was the head of the family; but in the meantime, my relationship with my mother would have become closer. She would have increased her protection, and I would have increased my incompetence. Although we, the family members, had other strings to our bows, in dysfunctional situations my family, like other families, would have used as its first strategies for problem solving its best-known solutions. And, of course, this more-of-the-same would have increased the homeostatic tendencies of the family instead of increasing its complexity and its capacity for new solutions.

Other families, though different in their idiosyncratic histories, share with mine the immediate homeostatic stubbornness as a response to stress. And although most families, as did mine, find a way out of crisis, a way of evolving into more complex problem solvers, other families fail and come to see a therapist. When they do, they present to the therapist their framing of the problem and their framed solution, and the therapist's framing will be different.

The therapist starts her framing by taking what the family considers relevant into account. But her way of gathering information within the context of the family already frames what they present in a different way. The therapist's task is then to convince the family members that reality as they have mapped it can be expanded or modified. The techniques of enactment, focusing, and achieving intensity are relevant to successful therapeutic framing.

In enactment, the therapist helps the family members to interact with each other in her presence, to experience the family reality as they define it. She then reorganizes the data, emphasizing and changing meaning, introduces other elements, and suggests alternative ways of transacting that become actualized in the therapeutic system. In focusing, the therapist, having selected elements that seem relevant for therapeutic change, organizes the data of family transactions around a theme that gives them new meaning. In achieving intensity, the therapist heightens the impact of the therapeutic message. She emphasizes how frequently a dysfunctional transaction occurs, the variety of ways in which the transaction occurs, and how pervasive it is in different family holons. Achieving intensity, like focusing and enactment, pertains particularly to supporting the experience of a new, therapeutic reality, where the symptom and the symptom bearer's position in the family are challenged.

7 Enactment

O Chestnut tree, great rooted blossomer,
Are you the leaf, the blossom or the bole?
O body swayed to music, of brightening glance,
How can we know the dancer from the dance?
                                        W. B. Yeats

In family therapy, Yeats' question is accepted as rhetorical: we cannot know the dancer from the dance. The person is his dance. Inner self is entwined inextricably with social context: they form a single unit. To separate one from the other is, as in Bergson's image, to stop the music in order to hear it more clearly. It disappears![1]

But the family members stop the dancing when they come into the session and try to describe, comment, and explain to the therapist how the music and the dance are at home. This limits the amount and quality of the information supplied to the subjective memory and the descriptive ability of the informants.

When the therapist asks the family questions, the family members can control what they are presenting. In selecting what material to communicate, they frequently try hard to put their best foot forward, as it were. But when the therapist gets the family members to interact with each other, transacting some of the problems that they consider dysfunctional and negotiating disagreements, as in trying to establish control over a disobedient child, he unleashes sequences beyond the family's control. The accustomed rules take over, and transactional components manifest themselves with an intensity similar to that manifested in these transactions outside of the therapy session.

Enactment is the technique by which the therapist asks the family to dance in his presence. The therapist constructs an interpersonal scenario in the session in which dysfunctional transactions among family members are played out. This transaction occurs in the context of the session, in the present, and in relation to the therapist. While facilitating this transaction, the therapist is in a position to observe the family members' verbal and nonverbal ways of signaling to each other and monitoring the range of tolerable transactions. The therapist can then intervene in the process by increasing its intensity, prolonging the time of transaction, involving other family members, indicating alternative transactions, and introducing experimental probes that will give both the therapist and the family information about the nature of the problem, the flexibility of the family's transactions in the search for solutions, and the possibility of alternative modalities for coping within the therapeutic framework.

When the family comes into therapy, there is usually consensus about who is the identified patient, what is the problem, and how this problem affects other family members. The members' prior attempts to find solutions on their own have centered their transactions too much around the "problem," making it the background against which all other aspects of their reality are played. Their experience of reality has narrowed down from overfocusing. The intensity of their experiences around the symptom and the symptom bearer has caused them to ignore other significant aspects of their transactions. The family has framed the problem and their transactions around the problem as the relevant reality for therapy. The therapist's problem is how to gather information that the family members do not consider relevant, and even more difficult, how to gather information that the family members do not have available.

There are a number of ways to solve this problem. Therapists who are trained to use the verbal, auditive channel of communication as the main source for gathering information listen to the patients, ask questions, and listen again. They pay attention to the content of the material elicited, to the ways in which the different elements of the plot relate with each other, to the qualifications of and the disparities between these elements, and to the affect of the presentation. This mode of gathering information cannot provide therapists with information that the family members do not have. A corollary of the therapist's over-reliance on content is a concern for completeness. The therapist tracks the patient, requesting further information on the themes that the patient has already presented as central, being careful not to intrude into the material, so that the history follows its own selective sequence. The therapist helps in the unfolding of the material until he has enough information.

This mode of inquiry preserves the myth of the objectivity of the therapist and the reality of the patient. The therapist is likened to an historian or a geologist trying to get an objective reporting of what is "really" there. This framing of the therapeutic process has developed therapists who hesitate to use themselves in therapy for fear of distorting the "reality," and they organize the therapeutic context into two separate camps: "they," the observed, and "us."

But therapists who have been trained in interpersonal channels of communication know that the act of observation influences the material observed, so that they are always dealing with approximates and probable realities. Dismissing the fantasy of an objective therapist and a permanent reality, the family therapist creates in the session an interpersonal scenario in which a dysfunctional transaction among the family members is played out. Instead of taking a history, the therapist addresses himself to bringing areas that the family has framed as relevant into the session. He assumes that since the family is dysfunctional only in certain areas, paying attention to these particular areas will provide insight into the central family dynamics. The assumption is that the family structure becomes manifest in these transactions and that the therapist will therefore catch a glimpse of the rules that govern transactional patterns in the family. Problems as well as alternatives thus become available in the present and in relation to the therapist.

When family members enact a transaction, the usual rules that control their behavior take over with an affective intensity similar to that manifested in their routine transactions at home. But in a therapeutic situation, where the therapist is in control of the context, he can test the rules of the system by affiliating differentially with family members or by entering into coalitions against other members. The therapist can also control time dimensions. He may say to the family members, "Continue this transaction," or he may block the attempts of other family members to shorten the enactment. In this process, the therapist attempts to change the affiliation of family members with each other temporarily, testing the flexibility of the system when the therapist "pushes." This maneuver gives information about the capacity of the family to change within a particular therapeutic system. Enactment requires an active therapist who feels comfortable with engaging and mobilizing people whose responses cannot be predicted. The therapist must be comfortable in open-ended situations, in which he not only helps to unfold data, but also creates data by pushing people and observing and experiencing the feedback to his intrusion.

Besides the improvement in the quality and quantity of the information provided, the technique of enactment offers other therapeutic advantages. First, it facilitates the formation of the therapeutic system, since it produces fast engagements between family members and therapist. Family members enact their dance in relation to the therapist, who is not only an observer, but also a musician and dancer himself.

Second, while the family is enacting its reality within the therapeutic context, there is a concomitant challenge to this particular reality. Families present themselves as a system with an identified patient and a bunch of healers or helpers. But when they dance, the lens widens to include not only one but two or more family members. The unit of observation and intervention expands. Instead of a patient with pathology, the focus is now a family in a dysfunctional situation. Enactment begins the challenge to the family's idea of what the problem is.

Another advantage of enactment is that, since members of the therapeutic system are involved with each other instead of merely listening to each other, it offers them a context for experimentation in concrete situations. This context is decidedly advantageous to work with families of young children or of children at different developmental stages, and with families of cultural backgrounds that differ from the therapist's. The utilization of therapeutic directives and concrete language and metaphors drawn from the transactions among family members facilitates communication across both cultural and age boundaries.

Although enactment occurs in relation to the therapist, it may also facilitate the therapist's disengagement. Families have great power to induce a therapist to function according to the rules of the family. They may triangulate him or force him into a centrality that robs him of therapeutic maneuverability. One of the simplest techniques to disengage is to suggest an enactment among family members. While the family members get involved with each other, the therapist can distance himself, observe, and regain therapeutic leverage.

Enactment can be regarded as a dance in three movements. In the first movement, the therapist observes the spontaneous transactions of the family and decides which dysfunctional areas to highlight. In the second movement of enactment, the therapist organizes scenarios in which the family members dance their dysfunctional dance in his presence. And in the third movement of enactment, the therapist suggests alternative ways of transacting. This last movement may give predictive information and bring hope to the family.

The three movements of enactment are illustrated in the treatment of the Kuehn family, the family who came to the clinic because Patti, age four, is a "monster." She is so uncontrollable that the parents have taken to locking her into the bedroom at night. Otherwise, she will run downstairs and light the stove, or run out into the street. The parents are at their wits' end.

The father, a burly though gentle and unassuming man, can control Patti adequately by himself. But his wife, a soft-spoken woman, is nonplused by her daughter. Patti is an alert little girl whose quick and lively temperament make her a striking contrast to her somewhat placid parents.

The family has been in therapy for seven sessions. The therapist's strategy for these interviews has been to have all of the family members present, including the two-year-old daughter, Mimi. But usually Patti and her sister have been sent to the playroom after disrupting the session, and her parents have remained to talk about their problem with her. In the eighth session Minuchin joins them as a consultant.

THE FIRST MOVEMENT: SPONTANEOUS TRANSACTIONS

Three minutes into the session, after the episode of joining reported earlier, dysfunctional family transactions are framed.

Patti: Is that mine? (*She takes Minuchin's papers*).
Minuchin: No! That's mine. (*Patti sits on the table.*)
Mother: Don't sit on the table, Patti. What is that?
Patti: That's the table.
Mother: Okay. Don't sit on the table, okay? You sit on chairs. Okay, honey?
Patti: Doc—doc—doc—doc— (*Continues to repeat this in the background as she runs around the room, hitting the back of each chair.*)
Mother: She seems pretty wound up lately. (*Mimi begins to follow Patti.*) No, Mimi. No, Sweetie.
Patti: I want to play with—here, Mimi, you play with the dragon. Do you have any paper?

Mother: No, not today, sweetheart. No, put that back, we don't have any paper to draw on. Put them back, Patti. Patti, do what you were told. Put them back. Her belligerence is so—

Minuchin: Is that how you run your life?

Mother: What's that?

Minuchin: Is that how Patti and you spend your time together?

Mother: Yes—yes.

Minuchin: It takes just a minute and a half to see it.

This episode contains all the information necessary for the definition of the problem. During this period, the mother makes seven ineffective controlling statements to Patti, whose amount of hyperactivity is matched by the mother's intensity of ineffective control. To the family's definition of the problem—that Patti is uncontrollable—can now be added another definition, that the mother is hyper-responsive in her controlling request, that her control is ineffective, and that she feels helpless.

Minuchin allows a spontaneous interaction between the family members to take place; this is essential to see how the family functions. Allowing such interactions to occur may seem like a simple thing, but it often proves difficult for the beginning therapist, who frequently confuses centrality with therapeutic power.

Mother: It's a continuous battle, at least for me.

Minuchin: Who wins?

Mother: It varies. If I'm up to fighting with her, at that point, sometimes I do. You know, I let her win sometimes, too. (*To husband.*) But we do try to get her to do what we say even if it is a fight. Don't we?

Father: I make her.

Minuchin (to father): What was your answer?

Father: I make her do it.

Mother: Right.

Father: I always win.

Patti (in the background): Doc—doc—doc—doc—

Minuchin: I feel there is a little difference there. You do make her, but your wife doesn't.

Mother: No, not all the time—no.

The definition of the problem is expanded here. The mother defines herself as understanding and helpless; the father defines himself as effective and authoritative; and they both define the daughter as uncontrollable. With this information, the therapist is ready to implement the enactment of a transaction around control.

The therapist guides his interventions here by a diagnostic assumption: When a preschool child cannot be controlled—when, in effect, he is taller than one of his parents, he is sitting on the other parent's shoulders. This diagnostic axiom, though not necessarily true with older children, seems to hold true with preschoolers. The parents can be expected to be in disagreement about the ways of controlling the child. The therapist does not yet know the patterns in which this dysfunction is expressed in this family, but he has all the information necessary to frame the area of control as dysfunctional, and to decide to bring that area into the session. He asks the family to take their usual steps to ameliorate the problem, thereby underlining dysfunctional transactions.

THE SECOND MOVEMENT: ELICITING TRANSACTIONS

Minuchin: Do you find this present arrangement a difficult one? For example, the two girls going around while we talk? How do you respond to that?

Mother: How do I respond to it? I get tense.

Minuchin: You get tense?

Mother: Yeah, I do get tense.

Minuchin: So, you would prefer that she stay in one place?

Mother: No, I can see them walking around when there are toys for them to play with.

Minuchin: What would you like?

Mother: Right now?

Minuchin: Yes, what would make it more comfortable for you?

Mother: For them to sit over there and play with the puppets.

Minuchin: Okay. Do that. Make it happen.

Minuchin tells the mother, "Make it happen." The stage is now set for a changed sequence of interaction. Rather than Patti and her mother playing their accustomed parts, in this scenario the script has been changed. The therapist-director has given the mother a new part: she will now act to get her four-year-old daughter to behave in such a way that the mother is more "comfortable."

By saying to the mother, "Make it happen," Minuchin has also conveyed an important message to her; that is, she is in fact capable of making Patti behave. It would have been quite different if he had said, "Why do you ask your daughter okay at the end of each command? Are you concerned with hurting her?" Both interventions, no doubt, would bring up information about the mother-child transaction; one, however, is a homeostatic maintainer, and the other introduces a destructuring challenge to the mother-child holon.

Mother: Patti, go over there and play with the puppets, okay? Go ahead. No, not here. No.
Patti: Why?
Mother: Go over and play with the puppets.
Patti: I don't love you.
Mother: I love you. Go ahead, go play with your puppets.
Patti: I don't want to play.
Father: Patti—
Mother: Mimi is playing with them—
Father: Patti, will you sit down? (*Speaks firmly and Patti looks at him.*)
Minuchin (to father): Let Mother do it. You know she's the one who does it when you are not there.
Father: Yeah, yeah.
Minuchin: So, let her do it.

When the family enacts a controlling transactions, the three members activate each other in their usual role function. The mother enacts her helplessness, and this activates the father to take over control, to be effective in his authoritarian style, so that the definitions of each family member in the family are confirmed. The daughter is impossible; the mother is helpless; the father is authoritarian. The therapist is interested in testing the limits. He wants to explore the flexibility of the family to function in unusual ways. Can the mother be effective in the presence of her husband? Can the father not be activated by his wife's momentary helplessness? Can Patti respond to her mother?

The rashness by which the therapist organizes this enactment may raise questions, and the creation of this scenario may seem rushed on his part, in contrast to a therapeutic strategy that gathers information in a broader area. The strategy of this enactment may indeed be criticized on two counts: the first has to do with the lack of historical information or even of transactional information about the family, since the therapist is just in the first six or seven minutes of the session with a family that he does not know. The second criticism has to do with the narrowness of the exploratory search. But the episode demonstrates a generic concept of gathering information. Through the process of creating a scenario, the therapist elicits information by pushing the family members against the thresholds of their usual transactions. The therapist then observes the response of the family members to this pressure. This is a transactional method for gaining information, in which the therapist gathers the information by experiencing the resistance of the family members to his prod. This technique makes for an immediacy of experience and gives a cross-sectional knowledge of the way in which family members function ordinarily, along with additional information on how they function when the therapist is producing pressures through his scenarios. This transactional information provides a biopsy of the family. The transactions as demonstrated by the probes are an experiential distillation of the family history. The advantage of the approach is that, in this small area, the therapist can gain an intensive knowledge of the way the family functions.

THE THIRD MOVEMENT: ALTERNATIVE TRANSACTIONS

Minuchin: Make it happen. What you said should happen. Make it happen. It's not happening.

Mother: Patti, what were you told to do? (*Patti whines.*) No. Go sit down and play with the puppets.

Patti: Come on, I want to play with this.

Mother: Okay. Play with that then, but why don't you try to play quietly, okay? While we talk. Okay? Go sit down with Mimi now. Pull up your socks.

Patti (pulling up her socks): These always fall. (*Both girls wander over to the mirror.*)

Mother: Sit down, Mimi. Get off that mirror, Patti.

Patti: Is this a mirror?

Mother: Yes. Don't touch it.

Patti: Now, Mimi, don't you dare. You daren't do this—you know what? The last time she caught her finger in the door and I caught my thumb—

Minuchin: It's not happening.

Mother: Well—

Minuchin: Find whatever way you need to, but make it happen. Organize the two girls to be in one corner playing so that you feel comfortable.

Mother: The only way I could do that would be to put them in a corner
with the—

Patti: Mimi, put that back!

Mother: —toys and me to stay with them.

Minuchin: Do it the way in which it is necessary for them to occupy
themselves and for you to be here with us. Make it a difference between the grownups that are talking and the children that are playing.
Make it happen.

Mother: All right. Patti, come here.

Patti: Doc?

Mother: Go ahead, sit down and play with the puppets.

Patti: I want to play with these.

Mother: Okay, sit down and play with them, then.

Patti (looking at the puppets): I can't find the woman and the little girl
and the baby.

Mother: Well, maybe someone else is using them today. Okay? There are
plenty of other toys over there for you to play with. Okay?

Patti: Okay, you play with this, Mimi.

In this segment there are four interventions by the therapist, all of
which represent a variation on the theme: it's not happening, make it
happen. The therapist, seated on the periphery of the scenario that he
has created, experiences the way in which the mother and Patti activate
each other, but he does not interpret or comment on what he is observing: the transaction between the girls; Patti's acting like her mother in
relation to Mimi or the mother's finding something wrong with the socks
when Patti does obey. His interventions are presented in such a way that
he maintains the members of the dyad working with each other around
the area of the enactment. An intervention that commented on the nature of the transaction between the mother and Patti would have induced the mother or Patti to establish a dyad with the therapist and
would have interrupted the mother-Patti dyad. The therapist is pushing
the mother and thereby gathering information about the flexibility of
the system to respond with his help.

The therapist then explores the possibility of the development of an
unusual transaction in this family, one in which the mother becomes ef-

fective in controlling the daughter without the intervention of the father.

Minuchin: Make it happen.

Mother: All right. Mimi, put that back. Patti, come here. (*Gets up, goes toward the girls, and takes a toy away from Patti.*)

Patti: Mimi gave the toy to me.

Mother: I know she did. Come on. I want you to bring all the toys over and play. Patti, bring all the toys over here.

Patti: Why?

Mother: You and Mimi are going to play. Okay?

Patti: Where?

Mother: Right here. (*Stands and ushers the girls into a corner.*) Right here. Why don't you play? Play mommy and daddy with the puppets and the baby. Okay?

Patti: Huh?

Mimi: I want a puppet, too.

Patti: Mimi, here's the father. In here are the two girls.

Minuchin: Very good. Now, relax—feel comfortable.

Mother: But, I know it is not going to last.

Minuchin: No—no, no. Relax. If you really feel that it will last, it will last.

Patti: Come on, Mimi, play. Come on, play. I want to take the cradle away.

Minuchin: You know, you have been successful at this point. The girls had a way of distracting you so that you say that something should happen and then you forget, and I see Patti being an experienced person in the distracting technique, you know, so that you are all the time busy with her.

The enactment of this situation finished with the mother being effective. Of course, this outcome is an artifact of punctuation. The therapist selects a moment at which the mother has been able, with his help, to organize the behavior of the two girls, and at this particular moment he declares the end of the enactment. The purpose of this strategy is to help the mother to experience herself as competent in the presence of her husband and in the presence of the therapist without the husband taking over or becoming authoritarian. The therapist assumes that it is possible for this mother to be competent with Patti, and he helps the family enact their reality with certain variations, since if the mother is effective, then the daughter's label of impossible will disappear as well.

In summary, the therapist remains peripheral so that interactions between the family members occur. Soon the problem appears. The therapist frames certain events enacted in the session, declaring them important, and encourages the family to ameliorate the problem, here and now. By blocking the father's entrance, he makes the usual end point impossible, forcing the mother and Patti to go beyond their accustomed patterns to the point where the mother actually asserts control. The therapist then labels her effort successful, underlining an experience of competence, and suggesting that change is possible.

Sometimes family members enter into transactions that the therapist can frame as highlights of their dance immediately. In this case, the first and second movements of enactment can be combined.

HIGHLIGHTING A SPONTANEOUS INTERACTION

The Hanson family consists of father and mother; Alan, age 19, who has been an inpatient in a psychiatric center for six months; Kathy, 17, who is close to Alan; Peg, 21, the parental child; and Pete, 12. The segment occurs within the first five minutes of the session. Minuchin, again acting as consultant, has just been introduced to the family.

Minuchin: Do you have a boy friend, Kathy?
Kathy: Yes.
Minuchin: Alan, do you have a girl friend?
Alan: No.
Minuchin: How long have you been going with him, Kathy?
Kathy: One and a half years, now.
Minuchin: My goodness. So, you started young. Alan, is her boy friend your friend?
Alan: Yes.
Kathy: He wasn't when I met him. I didn't meet him because he was Alan's friend.
Minuchin: But at this point, Alan, he is your friend. What is his first name?
Alan: Dick.
Minuchin: How old is he?
Kathy: Nineteen—
Alan (answering simultaneously): I don't know—nineteen?

Minuchin: You are helpful, Kathy. I asked Alan how old Dick was, and while he was thinking, you said nineteen. She didn't wait for you to ask her, Alan. She volunteered. Is that something she frequently does?

Alan: Yes.

Minuchin: Anticipating you?

Alan: Yes.

Minuchin: So, she takes your memory.

Alan: I guess so.

Minuchin: Who else in your family acts like Kathy? I saw your mother with Pete, just outside. Pete wanted to go to the bathroom, and your mother almost entered the bathroom with him, as if he couldn't find the men's room by himself. Did you notice that, Pete? Did you notice she went half of the way with you?

The therapist notices that Kathy first amplified Alan's statement and then anticipated and preempted his answer to the question about Dick's age. Adding an isomorphic transaction that he observed between the mother and Pete, the therapist frames all of these transactions as a family pattern that handicaps the individuation of family members.

Again the speed with which the therapist interprets such scanty data may raise a question about his reliability. It is also true that highlighting a dysfunctional transaction so early in his contact with the family might upset them. But the therapist's intervention is soft, supportive, humorous, and oblique, allowing him to join the family at the same time that he frames a dysfunctional pattern.

Having recognized the intrusive quality of the family's transactions and hypothesized that this is a central issue in the family, the therapist continues to underline intrusive transactions. The next segment occurs fifteen minutes later. The therapist directs Alan to change seats with his mother so that he can sit next to his father and discuss a problem. Alan moves, and then reattaches his lapel microphone. His father reaches over, picks up the wire that is draped over the chair, and moves it for Alan.

Minuchin: I want to show you, Alan. (*Gets up, stands in front of father and son, takes the cord, and reproduces the father's act.*) Your father took the cord and moved it over. Why did he do that? What was he doing?

Alan: I don't know. Trying to correct something, I guess.

Minuchin: Do you have two arms?

Alan: Yes.

Minuchin: Do you have two hands?

Alan: Yes.

Minuchin (taking Alan's arm): This arm finishes in a hand. Could you do that? (*Puts the cable from the original position to the place where father had located it.*)

Alan: Yes.

Minuchin: At nineteen, I assume, you can do that by yourself?

Alan: Yes.

Minuchin: Why did he do that? Isn't it strange that he should do that, as if you don't have hands?

Alan: Well, he does that a lot.

Minuchin: How old do you think he thinks you are? Three? Seven? Twelve?

Alan: Twelve.

Minuchin: So, that makes you a little bit younger than Pete. Can you help him? Can you help him so that he grows up—so that he lets you use your two hands?

Alan: I don't see how.

Minuchin: Well, if you don't help him to change, you will not be able to use your hands. You will always have ten thumbs—you will always have two left hands—you will always be incompetent because he is doing things for you. He is paralyzing you. Talk with him about that, because I think that's very dangerous what your father did just now.

The therapist balloons a nonevent into a moment of drama. An automatic, helpful movement of the father is framed as the spontaneous enactment of a dysfunctional transaction that is seen as isomorphic to the previous ones. This technique of framing a spontaneous and unattended event usually gains salience, since the family members are surprised when their attention is called to the fact that they are acting unwittingly and frequently in conflict with their wishes. In this segment, the therapist increases the intensity of the intervention by standing close to the dysfunctional dyad, by affiliating with Alan, and by using a series of concrete metaphors about individuation and coping. He finishes this maneuver by suggesting the enactment of a change in the father-son transaction in which Alan, who is always in a position of incompetence, becomes the father's helper.

Now the therapist begins to enact alternatives in this family. The first time, the family rules prevail.

Alan: Well, I think I know what he means, like sometimes—

Father: I know what he means, too, Alan, and it's the truth.

Alan (to mother): He does things for me.

Minuchin: Go beyond that, Alan. I think your father needs help, and I don't think that anybody can help him in that better than you.

Alan: I don't know what to say.

Minuchin (to Alan): I am a stranger, you see, and I can't help because I don't know you two. If you need some help, you can ask someone in the family to come and join you, but if you don't need to, I want you to try first by yourself.

Father: Do you want Peg to help you?

Minuchin (to father): Why did you select for him? Why did you select for him? You just now did exactly the same thing. You see, Alan, he is so absolutely hooked into being helpful that he cannot help himself. Now I want you to think if you really want Peg to help you or anybody else—or nobody.

Father and son activate each other's complementarity: Alan's hesitation calls forth the father's helpfulness, which is also control and intrusion. The father's helpfulness maintains the son's incompetence. The dysfunctional transaction is maintained. The therapist now has information about the level of rigidity of this subsystem. He knows experientially that at this juncture, his participation alone is not sufficient to introduce alternatives. He must change strategies or bring up reinforcements. He can have one or more family members join the dysfunctional dyad; he can maintain the same frame but explore it among other family members; or he can shift attention to a different aspect of the family dynamics and return to the same issue later on at a point where he finds himself in a more powerful position within the system.

Not all families plunge into their usual transactions with such alacrity. The therapist may have to take a position of leadership, asking questions and activating individual family members, in an attempt to get things started. In some cases, family members may remain guarded, trying to preserve their public image. But because the therapist is present in the room and transactions are related to him, he can increase the intensity by selecting certain parts of the transaction to highlight or by suggesting a continuation of the enactment in the same or unusual ways. The therapist can determine the parameters not only of the problem as it exists but also of the alternatives available, testing the flexibility of the system and gathering predictive information about the possibility that this family can function in different ways.

In some families the first two movements of the dance of enactment are quite easy to elicit, but eliciting transactions in an unusual way is not, because this movement requires an active participation on the part of the therapist in affiliation with some member before it is possible to determine what alternatives are available to the subsystem.

The Gregory family consists of a mother in her mid-twenties and her five-year-old daughter, Patrice. As in the Kuehn family, the mother is unable to control her daughter, but she is also afraid that she might physically harm her when she gets angry. Fifteen minutes into the second session, the girl is hanging onto her mother and not responding, in spite of numerous requests from her mother to sit quietly.

Minuchin (*to mother*): I think that Patrice has a way of making you dance to her tune. (*Patrice gets up and starts walking around the room.*) Tell her to stay there because I'm going to talk to you.

The therapist creates a scenario where he assumes that a controlling transaction will need to occur. He can use any number of simple situations, like this one, as a context where the family members are forced to enact their transactions. The simplest situation would be to have the parents ask their young children to do or not to do something different from what they are doing.

Mother (*in a soft voice*): Patrice. Patrice, come over here and sit down. (*Repeats it louder, since Patrice did not respond the first time.*) Patrice, come over here and sit down!
Minuchin: I like that tone of voice. That is your music. (*Patrice comes and hangs on to mother.*) You see what she's doing now? She knows your number and she makes you dance.
Mother: Sit down, Patrice.
Minuchin: Patrice has absolute control over you!

The therapist, who has joined previously with the mother in an affiliation of adults, challenges the mother to take an executive position.

Minuchin (*standing up*): Mrs. Gregory, can you stand up? Have Patrice stand next to you. See, Patrice is much smaller than you. Can you pick her up? (*Mother picks up Patrice.*) And you're stronger also. (*To Patrice.*) Hold my hand, tight. Let's see how strong you are. Very tight. (*To mother.*) Can you do that with my hand? No doubt you are stronger than she is.

The therapist uses a number of concrete operations designed to highlight the difference in power and function between parent and child. He expects this operation to unbalance the system, stressing the mother to join with the therapist and distancing her from her young daughter.

Minuchin: So, how is it that she controls you? (*Patrice again puts her arms around mother and hangs on to her.*)
Mother: Stop! (*No response.*) Stop it! (*Disengages Patrice and tells her to sit in the chair. Patrice obeys.*)
Minuchin: She needs to hear that voice. This voice is necessary. You are afraid of your stern voice, but this voice is good. At times it's soft and loving and at times it's strong, and she needs to hear both ranges. She needs to dance to your music.

The mother enacts effective control within a context in which the therapist supports her and puts the daughter down. This maneuver tends to be distasteful for many therapists, and it is so for the therapist in this session. But it is necessary to create distance between the members of this overinvolved dyad, to avoid the danger of child abuse, and to support the development of autonomy in Patrice, even in an aesthetically distasteful operation.

The therapist's behavior in this transaction is very different from that in the Kuehn family. There his participation is minimal, which facilitates the enactment of a functional transaction between mother and daughter. In the Gregory family, the mother needs the therapist's participation as an active member of the therapeutic system before enacting an alternative transaction.

A "HOW-NOT-TO-DO-IT" EXAMPLE

The Adams family consists of 24-year-old mother and her two children, ages eight and five. The problem is that five-year-old Jerry is abused by the mother. The mother at times loses her temper and beats him severely. The mother has referred herself to the therapist because she is concerned that she might harm her son. This is the initial interview.

The family enters and sits down. The eight-year-old, Molly, goes to the corner and quietly starts coloring. The boy immediately walks around the room, starts shouting, and gives his mother numerous commands. The mother, for her part, gives the boy various commands, such as, "Sit down and be quiet" or, "Don't say a word." After giving each of these commands, the mother quickly loses interest and does not follow through, even though the boy does not seem to hear her. At another time, the mother tells the boy to do a puzzle by himself. The boy takes the puzzle and hands it to the mother, who absent-mindedly completes the puzzle.

As the interview continues, the boy commands most of the mother's attention and scarcely lets her either talk to the therapist or attend to the girl. For most of the interview, the boy hollers so loudly that the mother and therapist can not hear one another. At other times, when the mother's attention is not directed toward the therapist, she is busy giving the boy numerous instructions. When the mother's attention is directed to the therapist, she and the therapist discuss such matters as how the mother can be more effective at home.

The only communication between the mother and the girl occurs at one point when the girl is busy doing a complete-the-dot puzzle. The mother looks down at the girl, sees that she is not doing it correctly and hollers at her, "You're doing your puzzle all wrong!" The therapist again captures the mother's attention, and they go on talking about how things can be better at home.

After about ten minutes, with Jerry grossly disobeying the mother, and the mother half-heartedly giving commands, the mother loses her temper. She hollers at the boy, gets up, grabs him, holds him by his waist so his head is hanging down unsupported, and brings him over to her chair. She then puts him on her lap, holds both his hands, at one point covers his mouth, and goes on talking. At this time, the boy is allowed no freedom of activity whatsoever, except breathing.

This session demonstrates a serious failure on the therapist's part. The therapist joins well with the mother and with the children. He speaks to the mother and joins with her around how difficult her life is. He speaks to the kids and has a similar rapport with them. He carefully observes the interactions in the family and notes a sequence of behavior that may and very probably does lead to the boy's being abused. He notes that the mother gives instructions and does not follow through on them. He notes that the mother either demands things that are inappropriately mature for a child of this age, such as sitting still and not moving, or ignores behavior that is grossly immature on the boy's part. He notes that the mother does not react immediately in an appropriate way to set limits for the boy. Instead, the mother waits and waits for her limit-setting to be obeyed. When it is not, she continues to wait, while the boy persists with his infuriating and antagonistic behavior. Suddenly the mother's threshold of patience is reached and she overreacts.

The therapist, noting all this, then tries to set up a situation at home where the mother can be a more effective caretaker. But instead of talking about the situation at home, the therapist could have realistically assumed that the sequence which transpires at home is essentially the same as what he has just witnessed. He could then intervene to change the way the mother and children interact in the session, with the sanguine assurance that the changed sequence would carry over to the home situation.

In order to enact a changed interactional sequence, the therapist could, for example, say to the mother: "You have a very high tolerance for noise from your children. It would help our work here if you could get them to be more quiet so we can talk. Do you think you would be able to do that?" If the mother says yes, then the therapist can say, "Fine, do it." If the mother says no, then the therapist can say, "Try, and I will advise you if necessary, but you need to do it."

There is a tremendous temptation on the part of the therapist to enter into a situation and produce the desired change himself. Had the therapist in this case said to the child, "Be quiet, your mother and I are trying to talk," he probably would have been effective to some extent, but the opportunity for therapeutic change would have been lost. The goal of therapy is, after all, to increase the complexity of the family's transactions and to facilitate their utilization of more competent transactions, not to develop a comfortable therapeutic holon.

This therapist lost an opportunity to turn the session from a therapy of history, cognition, and affect into a therapy of experience. Much vitality and intensity were therefore lost. And with a problem as severe as child abuse, the therapist needs all the intensity and leverage possible.

These examples of therapeutic sessions might give the impression that enactment is used only to create the major brush strokes, but this is not the case. Enactment is ubiquitous in all the small strokes, the small interventions that are repeated countless times in the course of therapy, such as blocking the mother and then listening and responding intently as the daughter finishes her own sentences, telling the teenage boy to negotiate with his father for the use of the car rather than letting his mother do it for him, or encouraging the parents to continue their conversation and not let their son intrude. Enactment is not a rarefied event that punctuates the course of therapy only occasionally. On the contrary, it should become a part of a therapist's spontaneous way of being, a pervasive attitude that insists on being there, when the family would be satisfied with just telling him what has happened.

8 Focus

Focus is a term borrowed from the world of photography, in which it represented a significant technical breakthrough. Early cameras only had pinholes. The photographer's emphasis was determined by where she was standing. If she was in front of the tree, the tree dominated the picture, even if William Howard Taft was standing next to it. The advent of lenses changed all that. The photographer could focus on a person, one flower in a bouquet, or even one petal. The relationship of the figure to the background could be controlled simply by making adjustments. Now the photographer could frame the world she wanted to portray.

In family therapy, focus can be compared to building a photographic montage. Out of a whole scene, the photographer decides that she wants to emphasize the house. Not the sky, the road, or the river; only the house. She begins to play with focus. She zooms in to make the door salient and takes a picture, then widens her focus to include the door and the window and takes another. She zooms in tighter, and shoots the doorknob. Out of this playing with multiple views of the same object, a multidimensional view emerges. It transcends mere description, to achieve the larger concept: the house.

In observing a family, the clinician is flooded with data. There are boundaries to be mapped, strengths to be highlighted, problems to be noted, complementary functions to be studied. The therapist will select and organize this data in some framework for meaning. But the organization ought also to be a therapeutic schema, one that facilitates change. The therapist will therefore arrange the facts she perceives in a way that both relates them to each other and has therapeutic relevance.

To do this requires, first, that the therapist select a focus and, second, that she develop a theme for work. At the same time, she screens out the many areas which, though interesting, do not contribute to her therapeutic goal at the moment. In the session, she selects elements of this family's transactions, and organizes the material in such a way that it fits her therapeutic strategy. By sifting out much of the information flooding her during the session, she is able to zero in on the data that are therapeutically relevant.

The therapist's schema includes both a structural goal and a strategy for achieving that goal. To challenge an extremely enmeshed family, for instance, the therapist may focus on the family's diffuse boundaries. How she does this will be determined by the content and process of the session. But the data will go through a transformation imposed by the therapeutic theme.

This is a hard lesson to learn. We humans are all content oriented. We love to follow a plot, and we are impatient to hear its end. But a content-oriented therapist can be trapped into operating like a hummingbird. Attracted by the many colors and tastes of affective disorder within the family, she flits from issue to issue. She gains a lot of information, satisfies her curiosity, and probably gratifies the family, but her usefulness in the session is limited to data-gathering. At its end, the therapist may find herself merely confused by the diversity of the issues. And the family may well experience the familiar discouragement of having told their problems to a therapist who "didn't help us at all."

By contrast, the therapist who develops a theme explores one small area in depth. Her data-gathering relates to the process of change, not to the family history and description. Instead of being transported from one plot to another while tracking the family content, she concentrates on a small segment of the family experience. And because family interactions tend to be isomorphic, exploring this small segment in depth will yield useful information on the rules that govern behavior in many other family areas as well.

There is an obvious hazard in focusing. The therapist develops a "tunnel vision," and she must be very aware of this. She must realize that once she has begun to develop a focus, she has programed herself. She begins to ignore information. Therefore, she must be supersensitive to warning indicators. She must hear the family if it tells her, "We are not following you." She must pick up feedback that tells her, "You are relating to your theories, not to us."

The therapist must also be aware that focus leaves her vulnerable to the dangers of induction. As she accommodates to the family and selects data, she may be seduced into selecting precisely the data that the family feels comfortable presenting. The therapist's job is to help the family change, not to keep them comfortable.

Jay Haley describes the case of a family with a drug addict.[1] The identified patient has been struggling to control his addiction and has been drug-free for two months. The family comes for the next session, agitated and depressed.

Father: We have a sad group here.

Mother: That's because I'm not coming back anymore. First of all, I'm moving. I am separating. Eric can go on his own. He's already made a mistake.

Therapist: You two want to separate? Is that it?

Father: I think it's the best thing.

Eric: I am the problem. You said you should go your way and she should go hers because I am a dope addict trying to make it.

The content of this transaction is an alarm bell to any therapist. But it is also, quite conceivably, a red herring. Therefore, the therapist in the case does not allow himself to be seduced into pursuing the content. He insists that the parents postpone any decision. In effect, he says that their separating is not relevant at this point. The three of them are in therapy to help the identified patient with his addictive problem. Because the therapist is following Haley's theoretical schema of how to work with drug addicts, he is able to decide to continue focusing on the chronic problems of parent-son transactions instead of the acute problems of husband and wife.

The therapist must sometimes postpone or ignore the exploration of both process and content material, no matter how tempting, to pursue her structural goal. She does not pursue her own agenda, heedless of its relevance to the family. But while paying attention to what the family presents, she clusters their data in ways that are relevant for therapy and decides on the hierarchical significance of those clusters.

PITFALLS

The Martin family was referred to therapy by the courts because the father, a nuclear physicist, had been sexually molesting his 15-year-old oldest son for two years. His wife of sixteen years had a good idea of what was going on, but she never confronted her husband.

The therapist begins work with several caveats in mind. He is especially concerned with avoiding a linear allocation of blame. The father has been abusing his child, but the wife has clearly been colluding, and by now the boy is a willing participant in the total process. The therapist also surmises that the husband's abuse of his son is at least partially an expression of problems between the man and his wife.

As a result, the therapist spends the early therapy hours dealing with the problems between the spouses. Since the family way of operating is to act as if the incest has not occurred and the spouses are quite willing to explore their difficulties as a way of avoiding the issue, the first few sessions are spent defining minor issues and helping the parents agree on them. At this point, the therapist and family are operating in a collusion of avoidance.

By the fifth session the supervisor suggests a reordering of therapeutic hierarchies. The therapist has to address himself to the child abuse rather than to the dysfunctional relationship between husband and wife. The therapist then enters the session and tells the parents: "You are a destructive family. I think you should consider whether you want to stay together, or whether you want a divorce." This question becomes the theme of the session. The couple now have to pull together to prove that they are not a destructive family. The problem affecting the boy is thus addressed, but in a way that also has the possibility of strengthening the parents' relationship.

The hierarchical reorganization of the family theme is another aspect of focus, for as the therapist highlights themes that she deems to be high priority, she often changes the family's idea of what is important. At times, the therapist focuses on a small moment of therapy and spotlights an interaction that is central to the family structure. The family, following her focus, experiences the transformation of the trivial and unremarkable event into a relevant theme. The very fact that the therapist has singled an issue out makes it important. The small, totally familiar interaction suddenly becomes unfamiliar; like breathing, it is only easy until you begin to think about it. From then on, the family reality that fit like an old shoe will pinch a little.

USE FOR CHANGE

In the Clatworthy family, the therapist weaves such small moments into a coherent theme. The family is composed of a single mother in her early thirties and four children: Miranda, age 13; Ruby, 12; and Matt and Mark, the twins, 11. Mark is the identified patient, although both twins are presented as a problem. They fight constantly, and they have been suspended several times from school for vandalism. The mother, who is on welfare, suffers from renal disease and hypertension; she has recently been hospitalized for gallstones. Both twins are eneuretic. Mark is in a special class; Matt is hyperkinetic. All the children have been suspended at one time and another, and they are regarded by the school as virtually uncontrollable. They are constantly threatened with foster placement by the mother and the agencies with whom the family is involved. The mother once placed the twins in foster care for a month, then changed her mind and brought them home, hoping to keep the family together. She came to therapy "as a last resort."

The family reality, as described by the mother, is characterized by constant fighting, lying, and stealing. She says that the children do not wash or change their clothes unless she does it for them. Ruby once took her menstrual pad off in public and threw it at a neighbor's house. The children defecate in each others' clothes, to get revenge.

The dysfunctional structure is a consequence of the hopelessness of the mother's world of poverty and debilitating illness and her own sense that she cannot cope with the demands of life, conditions which are exacerbated by the demands of the agencies that regulate the lives of the urban poor. All these factors organize her to look at her children with an emphasis only on deficit. Within the family, boundaries do not differentiate sufficiently. The mother and the outside agencies lump all the children together as one mass of problems.

Since the social welfare institutions emphasize only a partial aspect of the family's reality—its deviancy—the therapist determines to focus therapy on another partial aspect of reality—the elements of competence in this family. The therapist challenges the distorted worldview that sees the children's relationship to each other, to mother, and to the school only in negatives. He focuses on the more complex reality, including the possibility of competence rather than the hopelessness of deviance, so that this family may be able to make it through the difficulties of their situation.,

After the Clatworthy family has been in treatment for several months, the therapist, John Anderson, asks Minuchin to see the family with him in a consultation. The goal of the consultation is to help the therapist pull the family members away from their insistence on negatives and move them toward actualizing their competence.

Minuchin: Have you been in this room before?

Matt: Not this one.

Minuchin: Okay, Now I want you to tell me, what do you see in this room that is strange?

Matthew: I see cameras.

Minuchin: How many cameras?

Matt: One, two—

Mark: I see microphones—

Ruby: I see one, two, three cameras.

Minuchin: Three cameras. How many microphones? How many—show me.

Mark: One, two, three.

Minuchin: Okay, there are three. Now, what else do you see in this room that is spooky?

Ruby: The mirror.

Minuchin: The mirror. What do you think about this mirror?

Matt: It's got no glass on it.

Minuchin: Do you know what a one-way mirror is?

Mark: No, I don't know.

Minuchin: Okay, come here, and I will show you. Do you all want to come?

Mother: No, I know how it works. I've been here before. (*Minuchin takes the children into the room behind the one-way mirror.*)

The consultant starts the session by joining with the children in an exploratory game. Behind the one-way mirror he continues the game of exploration, turning the lights on and off and showing how the direction of the one-way mirror can be reversed. The children's response is curious, alert, interested, and participatory, and their comments are intelligent. Since none of these characteristics are included in the family description of the boys, the consultant feels inclined to explore this unacknowledged part of their behavior as a challenge to the concentration on their destructiveness by the family and the school.

The session is led by the therapist for the next fifteen minutes. The family is told that in this way the consultant will be able to see how the family and therapist dance together. During this period the mother complains to the therapist about the twins' behavior, while they express a curiously polite agreement with her. After fifteen minutes, the consultant takes over, while the therapist moves his chair back, indicating a change in leadership.

Minuchin: Okay, I am a little bit confused. Let me tell you what I saw. (*To children.*) I see that you are very bright and very observant. You enter the room and, just like lightning, you saw everything. So I see that you are very bright kids. I also see you work well together. I hear you talk, and you sound polite and bright and soft, and so I asked myself, "What's the problem with this family?" But maybe you have changed a lot in the last couple of months since you have been in therapy? Is that what happened? Is it possible, Ruby, that in the last two months you have changed completely?

Ruby: Probably so.

Minuchin: That's beautiful. Who else has changed? You, Mark?

Mark: No. Thirty-five percent has changed.

Minuchin: What is the way in which you have changed? This thirty-five percent, what is it?

Mark: Well, I wear underwear. I wear socks. I'm trying to make myself be smarter and everything.

Minuchin: And what about you, Matt? When your mother says that you were looking like bums, what does she mean?

Matt: She means that our clothes are dirty, our socks are mismatched.

Minuchin (*indicating the boys' present attire*): That means that you don't usually dress like that?

Mark: No, today I tried to get myself neat.

Minuchin: What about you, Matt? Would the teacher complain if you come dressed like that? How do you dress usually?

Matt: Sometimes I don't wear underwear—sometimes no socks.

Minuchin: And what is the problem with you, Ruby?

Ruby: Sometimes I wasn't doing my hair, and I wasn't wearing socks, or I used to wear dirty socks.

Minuchin: Then I am confused. You know, I really need a little bit of help, because you seem to be a very nice girl, a thoughtful and respectful child. So why don't you do what they expect from you?

Ruby: I just don't want to do it.

Minuchin: And Mother tells you that you should wear different clothing?

Ruby: She would say, "Wear the proper clothes."

Minuchin: And what would you say?

Ruby: I would just pay her no mind.

Minuchin: So, you are fighting with Mother. Not a real fight, but one in which you do whatever you want. Is that it?

Ruby: Yes.

Minuchin: Miranda, you are thirteen and you are the oldest. And you also look to me like a very well-put-together girl. What kind of issues did you have with Mom?

Miranda: Sometimes when she goes out and I see her house messed up or something, I do Ruby's job, or the twins' job. She'll tell me over and over again, "Don't do their job," and I don't pay her any mind. I just go ahead and do it.

There is a disparity between the children's demeanor, which is polite and cooperative, their dress, which is clean, neat, and esthetically pleasing, and their description of themselves, which emphasizes negatives. Even Miranda, the parental child, who has taken over many responsibilities because of the mother's illness, presents her responsible behavior in a negative framework. This single-parent family with a sick, depleted, hopeless mother has developed a structure in which the mother delegates functions to the parental child, but since the mother feels that it is wrong to do so, and that this constitutes a failure in her maternal role, she communicates a negative affect to a necessary structure.

Various social institutions support a negative framing for this family's reality. The Department of Welfare has threatened to cut off their income if the mother's boy friend of the past two years moves in with the family. The school sends continuous messages home about the teacher's difficulty with the twins, which frames the school problem as the mother's failure. And the therapist has focused on exploring the difficulties of control in the family and emphasized the mother's need to increase her executive functions.

The consultant, impressed by the general insistence on negative framing, is attracted by the family members and can spot positive qualities in their transactions. All of this reinforces his first impulse to challenge the family framing.

Minuchin: That means this house has two mommies?

Miranda: Um-hum.

Minuchin: Her and you? So, you are the good one. You are the responsible one.

Miranda: Not really.

Minuchin: I know that Mom is sick; and so, Miranda, you take over a lot of the things to help her.

Miranda: Yes.

Minuchin: And is it possible— I will ask you, Ruby. Is it possible that

you don't like it when Miranda acts like a second mother? Is she very
bossy?

Ruby: Sometimes she is.

Minuchin: And do you like that?

Ruby: No, sir.

Minuchin: When Miranda is bossy, what do you say to her?

Ruby: When she tells me to do something, I tell her to mind her own
business or get out of here or something like that.

Minuchin: So, you have a problem here between Miranda and Ruby.

Mother: I've always had a problem with them. I even had them separated for a while. Ruby is more introverted than Miranda. Miranda is
outgoing and tomboyish. She used to be very tomboyish. Ruby used to
be more domesticated and always playing with tea cups and dolls and
everything, but she's been with the boys longer. And Miranda stays to
herself a lot more than she used to.

The mother's description is highly differentiated; she is clearly a sensitive person who is observant of the children's individual developmental
processes.

Minuchin: Brioni, you will need to explain to me. I think you have very
beautiful children.

Mother: I do, too.

Minuchin: So, I don't understand. You see, I see them as beautiful and
bright and respectful so I am just confused. What are you doing in a
child guidance clinic?

Mother: Well, maybe because you're not with them all the time. The
teachers aren't saying they're respectful. Mark got suspended from
school last week for beating and stomping on his teacher, taking books
out of class—

Minuchin: Hold it a minute. I am confused. Mark, Mom says that you
are a terror in school. Is that true?

Mark: Yes, sir, I am.

Minuchin: So that means you are just conning me when you said, "Yes,
sir." And you act like you are really respectful, and in school you are a
terror.

Mark: Yes, sir.

Minuchin: What do you do in school?

Mark: I destroy school property.

Minuchin: You destroy school property? What does that mean?

Mark: It means that last month—

Mother: Last week.

Mark: Last week, I destroyed the boys' bathroom door and I destroyed the—

Minuchin: Why did you do that?

Mark: Because I didn't feel like opening the door, and I just kicked it and I cracked it.

Minuchin: That means you are a con man. I see you so polite and bright and kind of very, very much an all-11-year-old, but all of that is just a facade. You really are a gangster underneath. Is that true?

Mark: I'm not a gangster.

Minuchin: What are you?

Mark: I'm a little boy.

Mark accedes to the mother's request that he describe his "monster" behavior, presenting again a duality between the described and the manifest behavior: a gangster versus a little boy. Since Mark's behavior contains both parts, it behooves the consultant to select which aspects he will focus upon. In accordance with the therapeutic goal, he begins to develop a theme.

Minuchin: Do you know that story of Dr. Jekyll and Mr. Hyde?

Mark: I never heard about it.

Minuchin: Okay, it's a story about a very nice and gentle man who takes a medicine and gets transformed into a mean, evil man. Didn't you ever see that picture?

Mark: I never saw it before.

Matt: I know what you're talking about now. A man will turn into a wolf or something like that.

Minuchin: Are you just like that—very nice and gentle and sweet and respectful and loving and suddenly a monster, Mark?

Mark: Yes, sir.

Minuchin: You are like that. And now you are the lovely part, and when you go away, you become a monster. Is that the idea?

Mark: Yes, sir.

Minuchin: What kind of potion do you take? Do you take special things?

Mark: No, I don't. No, I don't take no pills or nothing.

Minuchin: And just on your own you become a monster.

Mark: Yes, sir.

Minuchin: Great! What a talent! Matt, can you do things like that?

Matt: I'm like The Hulk. When I get mad, I turn into a monster.

Minuchin: You also can change. Do you take any pills to change?

Matt: No.

Minuchin: Just on your own?

Matt: Just take your strength to change, that's all.

Minuchin: And you become a monster in school?

Matt: Yes, sir.

Minuchin: And at home, do you sometimes become a monster?

Matt: I never talk loud to my mother. I may get mad at her, but I don't call her names or anything.

Minuchin: Most of your monster act you reserve for school?

Mark: Yes, sir.

Matt: My mother said I won't be a survivor.

Minuchin: Why does she say so?

Mark: I don't know.

Minuchin: Can you ask her why she says so?

Mark: Yes. Why do you say I won't survive?

Mother: Because he's always manipulating people, beating them up, and it seems like he gets a high just manipulating people. And I've been telling him, one of these days I'm looking for somebody to knock him down from being a survivor.

Minuchin: I just want to tell you kids something. You know, your mom tells me bad things, and you are telling me that you become monsters, and so on, but I am mostly impressed by how bright you are.

Mother: Yeah, he's bright all right.

Minuchin: I am mostly impressed how clever and thoughtful you are. I am impressed with your brain.

By introducing the Jekyll and Hyde story, the consultant is accepting the family frame of the boy's destructiveness, but also expanding it to include the possibility of other transactions. Again, he focuses on the competence of the children.

Mother: Take him home. You'll find out.

Minuchin: No, I prefer them when they are the nice part of themselves. I am not interested in living with monsters. I like the way in which you are now. You are lovely.

Miranda: They are the same monsters—animals, too.

Matt: Like you are!

The mother challenges the consultant's emphasis, and this is a signal for the reappearance of the "correct" family behavior, a response that is designed to convince the consultant and the family that the consultant is, if not blind, at least myopic.

Matt (getting up threateningly): You're a zombie.

Minuchin: Are you going to give me a little bit of the act? Can you become a monster so that I can get a feeling?

Mark: I can't turn into nothing.

Miranda: Just ask them to get to fussing and fighting with one another and you'll see.

Minuchin: Hold it, Little Mom! Let the big Mom do it. Brioni, can you help them to become monsters so that I can see it?

Mother: The windows got broke Sunday when Mark tried to throw Matt out the window. *(Mark gets up and pushes Matt, who pushes back.)*

Minuchin: You're doing fine. You're doing fine. Make them do their act. I'd like to see it.

By asking the mother to help the twins become monsters and by making it into a game for 11-year-old children, the consultant emphasizes the possibility of control and self-control, keeps the focus on the interpersonal nature of behavior, and brings levity to an overheated area.

Mother: Well, Matt and Mark, every day they're fighting. At least once a month one of them is suspended. The school is telling me—

Matt: I didn't get suspended at all this month.

Mother: Not this month, but you were suspended last month.

Matt: For what?

Mother: Matt, you were suspended for hiding in the bathroom for a whole week, cutting class for a whole week.

Matt: But I didn't get suspended.

Mother: The problem with them is that they're slick. They know the rules and regulations of the school—what they can do and what they can't do—and they're using it to their best advantage.

Minuchin: That means that they are very bright.

Mother: The teacher told me they are too bright, but they're bright in a negative form. She said they're bright, and she said they're always trying to make somebody think they're being martyred, that somebody's picking on them. She said the principal will be so glad when June ends and they can get these twins out of this school.

At this point in the session an argument has developed between the consultant and the mother, since his emphasis is challenging the way in which the family members experience their reality. The consultant has become stubbornly wedded to the theme of competence and wants to "convince" the family members of the possibilities of an alternative framework.

Minuchin: Tell me, who is the better monster?
Mother: They can answer that. (*The boys begin to fight.*)
Mark (*pushing at Matt*): You don't have to stop.
Matt: Shut up, or I'll bop you in the mouth.
Minuchin: That's good. Go ahead. I want to see the monster act. Don't
  stop now. (*The boys start pushing and shoving, first lightly, but the
  intensity of their fighting increases.*) Okay. So that's how you are
  when you are a monster. That's excellent. And you do that frequently?
  At least I know now. So, that's their monster act.
Mother: Worse. That's a mild form of it.
Minuchin: Okay, so now you have two kids who are beautiful, bright,
  handsome, and—
Mother: I wish they had handsome behavior. I'd rather have ugly looking children and have children that at least act like human beings.
Minuchin: Hold it a minute. You see, you have two kids who are half
  beautiful and half monster, and they just happen to show more frequently their monster part. (*To the children.*) I am impressed with
  how bright you are, and also I saw a little bit of your act, and I think
  that you do it very well. Like two gangsters, looking mean like you are
  going really to kill each other. That was very good. Now what happens
  with Ruby and Miranda? Are they helpful?

The family is clearly puzzled at the consultant's lack of response to the reality that they perceive, and he has been receiving messages that he had better accommodate to them, or he will not have much leverage as a leader. He therefore changes his focus, moving to the behavior of the girls.

Mother: Miranda and Ruby are scared of the boys. When the boys get to
  arguing and fussing, the girls go somewhere and hide. Ruby will be
  with them more; Miranda will stay to herself. She's getting to the
  point now where she just ignores them.
Matt: We aren't the only ones in the house that fight.

Mother: I didn't say that, Matt.

Minuchin: Matt and Mark, do you gang up together against Ruby? Do you fight against her together?

Mark: I fight her by myself if she gets in my way.

Minuchin: Is he stronger than you, Ruby? You look like a strong girl. You are very tall.

Ruby: He's stronger than me. Sometimes Mark starts punching on me, and then I hit him back.

Matt: Tell him what you did yesterday.

Ruby: What did I do yesterday?

Minuchin: Hold it a moment. Hey, Matt, are you your brother's keeper? You see, just now she was fighting with Mark, and you entered to defend him. So, you work together.

Matt: Some of the time I don't.

Minuchin: That's what you just did. I think it's nice. Twins should work together.

Matt: I just told her, "Tell him what you did yesterday."

Minuchin: You were defending Mark. I see that you are on Mark's side.

When Matt intervenes, the consultant considers two options: he could maintain the boundary between Ruby and Mark, insisting on the need for dyadic transactions in an enmeshed situation. This intervention, while correct in the long perspective of treatment, would not be related to the present theme of positive alternatives. The consultant decides instead to emphasize the collaborative aspect of the transaction, transforming a usual gang-up in a sibling argument into a positive transaction. At this point the television camera moves, and the boys ask questions about the functioning of the camera. The consultant answers their questions and again focuses on their curiosity and competence.

Minuchin (to mother): I think that these are bright and exploratory children that somehow or other missed the boat and are thinking that the best part of them is the Mr. Hyde part. *(To the children.)* Even though you show me your monster act, I am still interested in the fact that you can be different.

Mother: They sure can. It seems to me that they go out of their way to do just the opposite. Even the teacher says they go out of their way to do what they want to do.

To the therapeutic organization of positives, the mother again brings the image of deficits, reinforced by the school labeling.

Minuchin: Mark, I am going to talk with Matt, and later I want your opinion. Okay? Matt, since you can be very gentle and bright and curious and you can also be a Mr. Hyde, an evil, monsterlike figure, I want to know what happens in the family, just in the family, that moves you from your angel face to becoming a devil. Who and what moves you from being an angel to being a devil?

The consultant takes the internalized label that has been programed by the family and the school and transforms it into an interpersonal issue, normalizing the monster.

Matt: Sometimes Ruby—
Mark: Miranda.
Matt: Sometimes she doesn't even mind her own business. She comes in our room every single day just to get her clothes, and she comes in there trying to be slick and saying, "Guess what you are in school," and she'll be easing her way in and we always tell her to get out, but she doesn't ever get out, so we go in her room and she says—(*The camera moves. Mark signals Matt to watch it.*)
Minuchin: Hold on! Did you notice also that while you are talking, Mark is helping you?
Matt: How?
Minuchin: Just a minute ago, when you were talking, he reminded you not to forget that the camera is following you. Continue, but I just wanted to show you that you two are really kind of nicely tuned in.

The consultant has two alternatives: to continue exploring the theme of the family as a context for the transformation of Mr. Hyde, or to focus on the support between the twins. He chooses the second alternative, building another element of the same theme.

Minuchin: So what you're saying is that you change from being nice to being a mean kid mostly when Miranda is turning you on. What about Ruby?
Matt: Um, Ruby doesn't give me cause.
Minuchin: Do you and Mark get on each other's nerves? (*Matt nods.*) You do. And then you can become mean also. So first is Miranda and then Mark? What about your mom?
Matt: Like yesterday, my mother wanted to be in her room and she doesn't like anybody in her room, and I was sitting in the hall and she

told me to get in my room. I got mad because I didn't do anything.

Ruby: Yes, you did. You got mad with my letter from my pen pal.

Matt: I didn't get mad over that.

Mother: Yes, you did. That's how it started. Ruby got a pen pal letter yesterday, and Matt got mad because Ruby wouldn't let him read it before she read it—

Matt: No, I—

Mother: Wait a minute, Matt. And I said, "Matt, when you got your pen pal letter, Ruby didn't read yours." He got so mad I had to ask Ruby to come in my room to read the letter because he wouldn't leave her alone.

Minuchin: I saw just now something important. You were talking, and then Matt wanted to jump in and you told him, "Wait a moment," and he did listen. Does that happen infrequently? Because just now you told him to stop and he did stop.

Again the therapist interrupts and establishes a point to build on the theme of competence. The focus moves to the mother and Matt's harmonious transaction in the area of control. Since the mother has been focusing only on her helplessness with the twins, the therapist brings this different transaction into focus.

Later, the consultant states a challenge to the family.

Minuchin (to boys): I just want to tell you again. You know, your mom and your sisters and the teachers all say that you two are monsters. I am a stranger, but what impresses me is your ability to reason, to think, to be thoughtful, to work together. I don't understand, because I am impressed with how good you are and everybody else is impressed with how mean you are. So I am very confused. You two confuse me and the school confuses me. Am I so dumb that the only thing that I see is the part of you that is nice?

Matt: If you were dumb, you wouldn't be here right now.

The therapist challenges the reality of the family, saying that there are aspects of themselves that are being short-changed. He joins and validates those unattended and unrewarded parts of the twins against the combined efforts of their significant others.

Mark: Shut up!

Matt: I can say anything I want to! Like, you behave like an angel? You aren't any angel.

Mark: I know it.

Matt: Then shut up!

Mark: No.

Miranda: It's only when you stay here, you're nice. When you go home, you act like animals.

Matt: Yeah, like you are.

Against the therapeutic framing of positives, the children bring back the focus on destructive competitiveness; but at this point the theme that the consultant has been developing is organizing his own perceptions and cognitive processes. This inductive process may be extremely helpful in therapy, because it helps a therapist to maintain focus. From the wealth of data he experiences, only those bits that are relevant to the development of the theme gain salience. So instead of being pulled or distracted by the routine truth of this family's competitiveness, which is irrelevant to the therapeutic goal, the consultant remains wedded to the theme of cooperation.

Minuchin: Matt, no, no, no. You see what she did just now? I am seeing the nice part of yourself, but she's not, because she knows the other part of yourself, and what happened just now is that she pulled out from you the mean part and you became mean. Did you see that? She laughed when I was saying you are nice kids. She laughed because she knows the other part of you, the Mr. Hyde, and immediately (*snaps fingers*) you became Mr. Hyde. (*To mother.*) You see, you have also done something for them that people do not tell you. You have been helping them to be curious. They are curious people.

Mother: I try to encourage them with books and things—take them to plays and libraries. Ever since they were little I tried to do that.

Minuchin: You have encouraged in them the ability to think. I just want to tell you, you have been very successful. (*Stands up and goes to shake mother's hand.*)

Mother (crying): You are the first one who tells me this. I see the positive side of them, but everybody else is telling me they are bad. The school board is telling me, "If you don't do anything about it, we will not keep them in school." It's hard to handle that all the time. I get tired of people telling me, "They're bad, they're bad." I know they're not that way all the time.

At this point the affect in the room changes. The consultant's support for the mother's efforts creates, for a small moment, a haven from the continuous criticism that she experiences. His acceptance of her efforts moves her to a recognition and support of the twins' unrecognized behavior.

Minuchin: Mr. Anderson, we will need to think together about how to help Matt and Mark get out of this rut because I see tremendous potential in both of them, because this mother has done a lot of things that she really does not acknowledge. You see (*to mother*), there is a lot of niceness in your family, and since you have been sick for a long time, there is a lot in them that is helpful and supportive.
Mother: Yeah, you know they can be that way. This has to be said, because I see the side of them that the teachers and people on the block don't see, and it makes it seem like I am looking—and they are telling me I'm looking—through rose-colored glasses.

At this point there is a neutral exploratory mood in the family members' transaction, and the session continues with an exploration of all the children's work in school. By the end of the session, the theme of Dr. Jekyll and Mr. Hyde has become part of the family's framing of the boys' behavior. This theme includes the idea of the good as well as the bad, but more important, it frames their "mean" behavior as part of the family transactions and gives the boys a tool for looking at their being a systemic "part" of the family organism. The therapist will need later on to deal with a whole series of significant issues that maintain the family dysfunctional transaction. But the focus on the boys' ability to use their Dr. Jekyll skills challenges the family's dysfunctional framing and gives leverage to the therapeutic system.

9 Intensity

A farmer had a donkey that would do anything he was asked. When told to stop, the donkey stopped. When told to eat, he ate. One day, the farmer sold the donkey. That same day, the new owner complained to the farmer. "That donkey won't obey me. When you ask, he will sit, stop, eat—anything. For me, he does nothing." The farmer picked up a two by four, and walloped the donkey. "He obeys," the farmer explained. "But first you have to get his attention."

Families are not donkeys any more than therapists are farmers. But the old joke has a familiar ring to therapists. In enacting the family scenario and in intervening to produce change, the therapist has the problem of getting his message across.

The therapist's intervention can be compared to an aria. Hitting notes is not enough. The aria must also be heard beyond the first four rows. In structural family therapy, "volume" is found not in decibels but in the intensity of the therapist's message.

Family members have a discriminating sense of hearing, with areas of selective deafness that are regulated by their common history. Furthermore, all families, even those consisting of highly motivated people, operate within a certain range. As a result, the therapist's message may never register, or it may be blunted. The therapist must make the family "hear," and this requires that his message go above the family threshold of deafness. Family members may listen to the therapist's message, but

116

they may not assimilate it into their cognitive schema as new information. If new information requires the acknowledgment of "difference," family members may hear what the therapist says as if it were identical or similar to what they have always heard in the family. Thus the therapist may have gained their attention, and they may even listen, but they do not hear.

Families differ in the degree to which they demand loyalty to the family reality, and a therapist's intensity of message will need to vary according to what is being challenged. Sometimes simple communications are intense enough, whereas other situations require high-intensity crisis.

The characteristics of the therapist are a significant variable in the development of intensity. Certain therapists can develop great drama with very soft interventions, whereas others require a high level of involvement to achieve intensity. Families also have different ways of responding to the therapist's message. Families who are ready for transformation may accept the therapist's alternative as a supportive push in the direction that they are willing to go anyway. Other families may seem to accept the therapist's message but in fact absorb it into their previous schemas without changing; while still others openly resist the change. A therapist who has been schooled to pay attention only to the content of messages may be so impressed by the "truth" of his interpretation that he fails to recognize that the family members have simply deflected or assimilated his message without gaining new information.

Cognitive constructions per se are rarely powerful enough to spark family change. Nonetheless, therapists are frequently satisfied that a message has been received just because it has been sent. But a therapeutic message must be "recognized" by family members, meaning that it needs to be received in such a way that it encourages them to experience things in new ways. Therapists must learn to go beyond the truth of an interpretation to its effectiveness. They can do so by actual observation of the feedback from family members, indicating whether the message has had a therapeutic impact.

Even when therapists recognize the ineffectiveness of their interventions and want to change them by increasing their intensity, they may at times be handicapped by rules of courtesy. Therapists, like their clients, have been trained since childhood in the appropriate response to people: respect and acceptance of their idiosyncrasies. Besides, therapists and family members belong to the same culture. They respond to the implicit rules of how to behave in situations in which people transact with other people. Therefore, when family members show in a session that they have reached the limit of what is emotionally acceptable and signal that it would be appropriate to lower the level of affective intensity, the therapist must learn to be able not to respond to that request, despite a lifetime of training in the opposite direction.

Once the therapist has observed a family's transactions and learned their accustomed patterns, the goal is to make the family experience the how of their interaction as the beginning of a process leading to change. The question is how to make the family "hear" the message. There are many techniques for making oneself heard.

Interventions for intensifying messages vary according to the therapist's degree of involvement. At the lower level of involvement are the interventions having to do with a therapy of cognitive constructions. At the higher level of involvement are the interventions in which the therapist competes for power with the family. In training, the middle levels of involvement are emphasized: the techniques of creating scenarios that increase the affective component of the transaction. These techniques may include a repetition of the message, repetition of the message in isomorphic transactions, changing the time in which people are involved in a transaction, changing the distance between people involved in a transaction, and resisting the pull of a family transactional pattern.

REPETITION OF MESSAGE

The therapist repeats his message many times in the course of therapy. This is an important technique for increasing intensity. Repetition can involve both content and structure. For example, if the therapist insists that parents agree on a set bedtime for their child and the parents have trouble arriving at a decision, then the therapist can repeat that it is essential for the parents to agree (structure) on a bedtime (content).

The Malcolms are the family who were referred for family therapy because Michael, 23, had been hospitalized for two months following a psychotic break during his senior year at professional school. During that period his wife, Cathi, lived with his parents.

At the initiation of family therapy, the young couple set a date to move out of Michael's parents' home into their own apartment. On the day of the move, with their new apartment entirely furnished, Michael slept until two in the afternoon. Cathi, testing her husband's commitment to her as compared with his loyalty to his parents, let him sleep. The session with the couple takes place the next day.

Fishman begins the session by asking why the couple did not move. The man lightly passes off his oversleeping: "We didn't move out because I overslept. I forgot we were going to move."

The therapist views the man's failure to move and his nonchalant attitude as a repetition of a life pattern that has organized him as controlled by the other family members—first the parents and now the wife. The move was something that had been planned for months. Furthermore, the couple and his parents had been busy readying the place for two weeks. For Michael to say blithely, "I forgot," is to abdicate responsibility for his actions while organizing the behavior of the rest of the family members. This is directly contrary to the goal of therapy, which is to increase Michael's autonomy and responsibility, so that he is not forced to use madness as a way of achieving desired change in his environment but instead can act directly, as a normal person, to produce whatever change he desires, whether it is to increase his closeness to his wife or to get out of an extremely tumultuous relationship. Either way, the normal behavior would be for him to take responsibility for the change, rather than to become symptomatic so that the changes in his relationship result only as a by-product of his madness.

The therapist, supervised here by Jay Haley, intervenes by asking Michael, in his wife's presence, why he did not move. At first Michael responds with vague answers in which he abjures any responsibility. The therapist then decides that increased intensity is necessary in order to get Michael to "own" his action. So he sets about asking Michael, repeatedly, "I wonder why you didn't move out." In the course of the session, which lasts about three hours, the therapist asks Michael about seventy-five times, "Why didn't you move out?" Michael continues to deny any responsibility.

The session lasts so long because the therapist needs to generate enough intensity to force the issue of why Michael has not committed himself either to living closely with his wife in their own apartment or to saying that he does not want to live with her because he is unsure about the relationship or unhappy with her. It takes three hours for both Michael and his wife to see the matter, not just as some anomaly that Michael did not get up in time to move out, but as a grave issue that is central to them both and which requires an answer.

As the session goes on, Cathi comes to regard her husband's failure to move out of his parents' house as more and more significant. She begins speaking of him as unable to leave his parents. Finally, she says that she wants to move out alone. Michael starts to cry: "No, I won't let you move out alone. I want to go with you." Cathi replies, "No, you didn't move when you had a chance, so now I'll go alone."

Michael is in a dilemma. To let Cathi move out alone would leave him home with his parents without Cathi to act as a buffer between him and his mother. Yet he cannot forbid Cathi to move. It is her apartment, too, and as she has the only job between them, she can afford to maintain the place. For the purpose of this particular therapeutic strategy, Michael is treated temporarily as if he were the beginning of the circle, or in control of the situation which clearly he is not. Finally Michael says, "Okay, you can move out." Now Cathi begins to indicate that she really does not want to move alone. Two days later, the couple move together to their new apartment.

Fishman here focuses on both structure and content to increase intensity. The content is, "Why didn't you move?" The structure is the powerful implication that Michael's decision not to move is tied to his relationship with his wife and parents. Evidence that the therapist's message has been effective comes from the fact that Michael makes a decision. He moves out with Cathi to their new apartment.

For the therapist to talk about nothing else for an entire session suggests that the topic must be very important. Furthermore, the therapist produces intensity in terms of process. If the therapist refuses to move, the family is forced to move; that is, there is a rearrangement around the static therapist. Patterns that in the past have been inflexible must now be modified in order to accommodate to the immovable therapist. Had the therapist allowed himself to be moved, he would have acted like the other members of the Malcolm family. In this family, all members have a lower threshold for modifying their behavior than Michael does. This allows Michael to remain static, while all around him change. By being unmoved, the therapist changes this pattern, forcing Michael to move.

The therapist can secure unwavering attention to a single issue by describing it again and again in the same phrase, like a litany. Or he can use a variety of ways to describe the same issue, using his capacity for metaphors and imagery like a poet or painter, focusing on a variety of transactions in such a way that every new description highlights the sameness of the transactions. Using repeated concrete images to give clarity and intensity is frequently necessary in working with families with young children and with retarded children or adults.

The Lippert family have been referred to the clinic because their 20-year-old moderately retarded daughter, Miriam, has anorexia nervosa.

During the six months of treatment, the family have done well. The parents have pulled together, and Miriam has gained weight as well as making progress toward becoming more autonomous. But in spite of Miriam's improvement, the family's attention has continued to be riveted on her eating. Their failure to leave this issue has made mealtimes the continued scene of a power struggle between parents and daughter. This past week Miriam lost four pounds. The family is very worried, and Sam Scott, the therapist, has requested a consultation.

The consultant decides to remove eating as a bone of contention so that the power struggle over it can stop. He tells the family that the issue of Miriam's weight will be between Miriam and the therapist, who will weigh her every week but tell the parents her weight only if there is cause for concern. Otherwise her weight will be her business, and the therapist will be the only other person to know what it is. Although the parents agree with the consultant, he knows from experience that he also needs Miriam's help to make possible the transactional change. This requires a systematically slow repetition of the message in terms that Miriam can hear and in such a way that it will also frame the behavior of the other family members.

Minuchin: Let's jump out of the groove. (*Touches Miriam's hands.*)
   Miriam, are these your hands?
Miriam: Um-hum.
Minuchin: They are not your father's hands?
Miriam: They are not.
Minuchin (*touching her biceps*): Is this your muscle?
Miriam: Yeah.
Minuchin: Are you certain?
Miriam: Yes.
Minuchin (*touching her nose*): Is this your nose?
Miriam: Um-hum.
Minuchin: Not your father's nose?
Miriam: Yeah.
Minuchin: Are you certain? Absolutely certain?
Miriam: Yes.
Minuchin: Is that your mouth?
Miriam: Um-hum.
Minuchin: Who eats when you eat ?
Miriam: Me.
Minuchin: Where does the food go?

Miriam: In me.

Minuchin (gently pinching some skin on Miriam's arm): Is this fat your fat?

Miriam: Yeah.

Minuchin: Yeah. So why do they tell you what to eat? Is it right that your father tells you what to put in your mouth?

Miriam: I guess it is right.

Minuchin: No. It's wrong. It's wrong. It's your mouth.

Miriam: Yeah.

Minuchin: Can you open your mouth? Open it. (*Miriam slowly opens, closes, then opens her mouth.*) Close it. Open it. Can you bite your lips? (*Miriam does this.*) It's your mouth. When you eat, will you eat by yourself the food that you want? And then when you come here, you will go with the therapist to weigh yourself. (*Picks up father's hand.*) Who's hand is this one?

Miriam: My dad's.

Minuchin: You are certain it's your dad's? (*Lifts Miriam's hand.*) And whose hand is this?

Miriam: Mine.

Minuchin: You are certain? Okay, so it's your body, you will feed it. How old are you?

Miriam: Twenty.

Minuchin: Does your father need to tell you what to eat?

Miriam: No.

Minuchin: Does your mom?

Miriam: No.

This is an example of increasing intensity by repetition of the content. The therapist, at the same time, asserts and reasserts the boundary between Miriam and her parents, challenging the family structure. The message is graphic, unambiguous, and powerful. In this example, gentle humor is used to make a high-powered point to a frail, retarded girl and a rigid family system. The humor adds intensity to the message.

A similar technique is used in the Hanson family when the therapist asks Alan if he has two hands. However, in that case, instead of accompanying the repetition with gentle humor, the therapist stands up, decreases the distance between himself and the father-son dyad, and adopts a serious tone of voice to convey that the situation is one of the utmost gravity. The same technique is used in a way that is appropriate for the particular situation.

REPETITION OF ISOMORPHIC TRANSACTIONS

A different kind of repetition involves messages which superficially appear varied (unlike the single "Why didn't you move out?"), but which are alike on a deeper level. Although their content is different, they are addressed to isomorphic transactions in the family structure.

Family structure is manifested in a variety of transactions that obey the same system rules and which are therefore dynamically equivalent. A challenge to these equivalent [*iso*] structures [*morphs*] produces intensity by the repetition of message in process. This intervention can focus on therapeutically relevant transactions and bring seemingly disconnected events into a single organic meaning, increasing the family members' experience of the constraining family rule.

In the Curran family, consisting of an enmeshed dyad—a widowed mother and her only son—the therapist makes various interventions. Fishman insists that Jimmy look at him and not his mother when they are talking. He encourages Jimmy to learn to drive and to start dating. He praises the mother when she mentions joining a Great Books group, and he convinces the two that Jimmy, age 18, should be able to sleep with his door closed and be responsible for waking himself in time for school. The content of these interventions is different, but they are structurally equivalent, and hence identical in process.

Single interventions, no matter how inspired, are rarely effective in changing patterns of interaction that have usually gone on for years. Systems have an inertia that resists change, and repetition is required for repatterning to occur. Therapy is a matter of repetition, in which desired structural changes are pursued in many different ways. The therapist's goal, new and more functional transactional patterns for the family, is kept in the therapist's mind throughout the session. It guides his repetition of therapeutically relevant interventions.

The Thomas family has been in family therapy for over six months because Pauline, 11, is asthmatic. Her asthma started when she was three years old, and during the last few years she has been hospitalized in intensive care as frequently as four or five times a month. The participants in the session are the mother, in her late thirties; Pauline; her brother, David, 13; her grandmother, in her early fifties; the mother's older brother Jim, who lives with his girl friend in the same house; and Tom, a younger uncle in his twenties.

The therapist, Kenneth Covelman, introduces Minuchin to the family as a consultant. Minuchin shakes hands with every member of the family. Pauline says that she does not shake hands. The consultant introduces himself to the mother, who shakes hands. Then Pauline says that she can shake hands with him also, which they do.

Mother: I don't usually shake hands, and I think she took after me.
Minuchin (to Pauline): How old are you?
Pauline: Eleven.
Minuchin: And you talk?
Pauline: Yes.
Minuchin: But your mommy talks for you sometimes?
Pauline: Sometimes.
Minuchin: Like just now?
Pauline: Yes.
Minuchin: Now, I will ask again the same question. Why did you shake hands with me now?
Pauline: Well—
Minuchin: Why?
Pauline: Because my mother did.

The therapist takes a small incident at the opening of the session and frames it in such a way that it becomes a significant event. The closeness between the mother and the identified patient is highlighted; the boundaries between the familial and the outside world are underlined; and at the same time, the therapist begins to focus on the identified patient, activating her. This small incident represents a theme that will be repeated throughout the session in a variety of isomorphic transactions, giving it intensity, until it is defined as the real problem in the family. The therapist begins to track this issue.

Minuchin (to Tom): I noticed how close Pauline is to Mother and how close Mother is to Pauline. Is that true in other situations?
Tom: Yeah. Even at home, they're very close.
Minuchin: To the point at which Pauline behaves like Mother behaves?
Tom: Somewhat, yeah. Because if, say, her mother's upstairs asleep and Pauline hasn't been downstairs for a long time and she hasn't seen her mother, or what not, she'll want to know if the mother's upstairs or did she go to the store, or vice versa.
Minuchin (to David): How old are you?
David: Thirteen and a half.

Minuchin: Is the situation between David and Mother different, or is it also close?

Tom: It's close. Not as close, but it's close.

Minuchin: Do you think that David is too close to Mother? As a boy of thirteen, do you think that he should be more independent?

Tom: Well, you know, he's basically independent, but he tends to stay close to his mother now, basically, because of her having a baby, and then, on the other hand with Pauline, because he tries to watch his sister.

Minuchin: His mother watches Pauline, and he also watches her?

Tom: David watches both of them. He tends to watch his sister a little closer because he, in a sense, can tell when she's having these attacks. 'Cause she won't say anything to anybody else.

Therapist (to Pauline): And you will tell your brother about your attacks?

Pauline: Sometimes.

Minuchin: Jim, what's our feeling about the question of closeness between Pauline and her mother?

Jim: They're very close. Sometimes their affection is a little bit too much affection.

The theme of the closeness between the mother and Pauline is expanded to a closeness between the mother and son and then to a closeness between the brother and sister. By tracking and questioning in a single area, family closeness, the therapist has moved very fast from the observation of one family member, the identified patient, to an elaboration of a problem that the whole family has. The mother then takes out something from her coat and gives it to Pauline.

Minuchin (standing up and walking over to Pauline): What did you just do, Mother?

Mother: Oh, I just gave her her barrettes to hold so I won't forget them because they were in my coat pocket.

Minuchin: What are those?

Pauline: Barrettes.

Therapist: I am looking at what is making Pauline have these attacks. I am watching how close, Mom, you are with Pauline. It seems, Mom, that you don't finish and Pauline begins, that you and she are like one body.

The therapist again takes an apparently meaningless incident that occurs in the transaction between mother and daughter and reinterprets that incident in terms of the closeness between mother and daughter. He is reinforcing a theme that he has constructed by utilizing observations of concrete events in which he and the family members have participated jointly and in the present. At the same time, the therapist is tying the observation of closeness to the asthma attacks of the identified patient. Ten minutes later, while Jim is telling about an incident in which he took Pauline to the intensive care unit, the mother begins to talk about Pauline's hairdo, and the therapist again focuses on this particular transaction as another instance of the mother's encroachment into the patient's self-definition.

Minuchin: What happened just now?

Mother: I asked her why she didn't have those rollers out before she came down.

Minuchin: And what did you say, Pauline?

Pauline: She said she was going to do it.

Minuchin: Did you roll up your hair?

Pauline: No, my mother did it.

Minuchin: Your mother. And you like her doing that?

Pauline: It's all right.

Mother: You don't like the way I roll your hair up?

Pauline: It's all right.

Mother: "All right" means you don't like it.

Minuchin: Ask again. Go ahead, Mom.

Mother: All right! Maybe it'll do, but it wasn't exactly put the way you want it, huh?

Pauline: It was put the way *you* wanted it.

Mother: Well, you didn't say anything was wrong when your hair was rolled up.

Pauline: Because *you* were rolling it up.

Mother (laughing): I'm going to punch you in the nose.

Pauline: No, you're not. (*Laughs.*)

Minuchin: No, no, no, no. This is not a laughing matter. This is important. It's important that you did let your mom roll up your hair the way *she* likes it and you didn't tell her that you didn't like it like that. Why didn't you tell her?

Pauline: Because she wanted to roll my hair up.

Minuchin: Yeah, but you don't like it. Okay, I am talking about Pauline having a voice and a mind and then having a body. If Pauline has a voice and a mind, then she will control her body.

While the theme in the session remains pretty much restricted to the nature of enmeshment in the family, the therapist centralizes the identified patient and works through her. His interventions are slow, accommodating to the lack of initiative of the identified patient, but insisting on a dialog with her that at times seems almost like an echo. The results of this type of support for the girl's initiative and of challenge to the family's enmeshed style of transaction are evident when the identified patient is able to challenge her mother. This change in the identified patient's style of transacting with her mother is feasible only because of the insistence of the therapist on the same theme for the last twenty minutes.

Minuchin: Now, be straight with me, Pauline. Do you like your hair like that?

Pauline: Yeah.

Minuchin: Are you certain? Are you certain that's what you want? Look straight in this mirror. It's not that Mom likes it like that?

Mother: Do you know what he means?

Pauline: No.

Mother: He means—

Minuchin (to mother): Hold it. Hold It. (*To Pauline.*) You don't know what I mean? I will tell you that. Ask me.

Pauline: I don't know what that means.

Minuchin: You still don't understand? Very good. Now, Mommy didn't talk for you, you talked for yourself. That's good. (*Shakes Pauline's hand.*)

Pauline: What did you shake my hand for?

Minuchin: Because I shake hands when I like something. That's my way of saying I like that. It's good that you're beginning to think separately from your mommy. Your mom is learning not to talk for you. And one of these days you will talk for yourself. (*To mother.*) Do you think she will be able to talk for herself?

Mother: I hope so.

Therapist: But, for Pauline to change, you will need to change.

The therapist is continuing the same theme in the same slow movement. The therapist is concrete and repetitive; he establishes contact with the girl at a very concrete level, which is necessary to activate someone who has been made the recipient of the family's support, protection, and control. When the girl fails to understand his statement, the therapist does not respond to her lack of understanding but instead interprets her request for information as an act of autonomy, confirming the patient instead of stressing her difficulties. In this episode, the therapist's use of isomorphic transactions gives intensity to his message that the pattern of overprotection of the identified patient is contributing to her manifest symptomatology. The technique that the therapist uses here is to work through the child, producing by his strategy an increase in the child's ability to initiate actions, request information, and differentiate herself from her mother.

Grandmother: I've had Pauline on the weekends with me, and she'd get attacks. Well, my nerves are bad anyhow, and this would scare me half to death, and I'd have to rush her to the hospital or call the police. But that's another reason why we've been so close to her. Now, what would be the cause of Pauline not to tell when she's coming with one of these attacks?

Minuchin: Pauline is here. Ask her.

Grandmother: Pauline, what is your reason for not telling us when you knew these attacks were coming on? Was it that you didn't want to go to a hospital and be stuck so much like they used to stick you?

Pauline: Yeah.

Grandmother: These needles would frighten you?

Minuchin: The thing that I'm trying to do here is for Pauline to learn to talk for herself, to think for herself, to feel what she feels in her own body. I think that because the family is so loving, Pauline is not caring for her own body. First you asked her, "Why do you get upset?" And then what did you say?

Grandmother: And then I asked her why she would tell us because—I said, "Why do you think, because the doctors are sticking you with these needles?" But she had told me that before.

Minuchin: You asked her a question and you gave her also an answer. So this young girl did not think. She did not think of it, because she could say yes, and that's it. And what I want to help you with, Pauline, is to think on your own, because in my experience—and I have seen many children with asthma—when children with asthma learn to have their own minds, a mind of their own, they also learn to control the asthma.

The mother's overprotectiveness of her daughter is presented as being repeated by different participants. The grandmother deals with the granddaughter by supporting her passivity and not requiring from her the kind of response that would be expected from an 11-year-old of normal intelligence. The therapist challenges the grandmother, who responds to the criticism with anger. Her mood then elicits nonverbal signals on the part of other family members which are supposed to instruct the therapist not to cross the grandmother. Yet the ability of the therapist to challenge the grandmother and maintain his position is an important example of differentiation for this family.

CHANGING THE TIME

Family members have evolved a system of notation to regulate the tempo and time of their dance. Some of these notes are conveyed by small, nonverbal signals that carry the message, "We have reached a dangerous threshold, or an unused or unusual pathway. Beware, slow up, or stop." This signaling is so automatic that family members respond without being aware that they have reached forbidden territory and have been brought up short by the reins of the family system. Like a well-trained horse, they respond before the rein is shortened and thus do not feel the bit in their mouth.

One of the techniques for increasing intensity is for the therapist to encourage the family members to continue transacting after the rules of the system have indicated a red or yellow light. Although the prolonged transaction is done hesitatingly by the family, their move from the habitual into the unfamiliar opens up the possibility of their exploring alternative modes of transaction. Similar results can be achieved by reducing the time in which people are usually involved in a transaction.

For instance, in the Kuehn family, after the family has transacted the steps that regulate their usual patterns for control, the therapist creates a scenario where the mother and daughter play with puppets making Christmas cookies. After a while, the father joins the game. This scenario is kept going for around twenty minutes, long after the family members indicate that they want to stop it. The long transaction around pleasure and nurturance involving the father as well as the mother carries in itself, without any verbal commentary by the therapist, the message of the unused but available possibilities in the family system: the father has the capacity for softness and nurturance.

In the Jarretten family, the therapist has difficulty in helping the mother and daughter to continue negotiating around issues of mutual respect as adults beyond their usual threshold of negotiation. The family comprises a widowed mother and her 18-year-old daughter Julie, who has left school in the middle of her first year and returned home. The mother and daughter are trying to work out some kind of coexistence.

Mother: I am changing my mind. I was not going to ask Julie for the money that I am giving her, but I am.

Fishman: I don't think you can change your mind every week.

Mother: If you want to kick us out, then kick us out. I am changing my mind as a result of her behavior.

Fishman: You let her down, too. You promised to pay her at a given time, and you promised that her money is to spend the way she wants to. I think the two of you have to work out a way. You are two adults. She is not your little girl anymore.

Mother: Do you know what the money is being used for?

Fishman: That's her business. She is not your little girl anymore. She is growing up.

Mother: She bleached her hair. All she uses the money for is for herself. The least I can get is a little respect.

Fishman: I want you to look at Julie.

Mother: I don't want to look at her. I'm tired of looking at her!

Fishman: I want you to do it anyway. Look at her. She is not a little girl anymore. She's very pretty. She's a grown woman. Now I want you to talk to her, not like she's a little girl, but like she's another adult living in your home. Because that is really how it is.

The mother and daughter's pattern of mutual negotiation is very short, interrupted whenever one of them stops it by introducing a complaint about the unfairness of the other. The therapist helps the mother and daughter to begin to negotiate issues within the frame of "mutual respect," and he frames the mother's beginning complaint in terms of a continuation of the same need for respect. He repeats and rephrases over and over the theme, "Your daughter is an adult, not a little girl." When the mother resists giving up her grievance, the therapist does not get involved with its content but simply repeats his message, "Treat her as an adult."

Mother: But she is not acting like an adult.

Fishman: I don't think this is Julie having a little girl's tantrum. This is a grown woman who had a contract with you.

Mother: I just don't want you hanging around the house and waiting for your boy friend. I would like you to get a job in the interim until you start school again—if you want to start school. (*To therapist.*) The reason I have been so inflexible is because I have made up my mind about something before we came in—

Fishman: Unless it is relevant to this topic, tell me later.

Mother: Okay, I will tell you later.

Fishman: Now, this is going to call for more flexibility.

Mother: I am sick and tired of this flexibility. I have had 18 years of this, and that is about enough. I don't want anymore. I want her out of the house. I don't want her in the house anymore.

Therapist: Talk to Julie about that.

The therapist resists the induction by other "juicy themes" that the mother dangles in front of him—"Unless it's relevant, tell me later"—and then activates mother-daughter transactions. His previous challenge to the mother gives the daughter space to respond to her from a position of being supported, which may allow for beginning of change in the transaction.

Julie: I want her to see my side. You said I could say my side—

Mother (*interrupting*): Julie, you—

Julie: I'm talking now. My boy friend and I were messing around in my room. I don't have to go into details to explain what we were doing, or how we kid around, or what kind of relationship we have. My mother knocked on the door harshly, and she embarrassed me no end. She said, "Bob, leave Julie alone, or I am going to beat you up." It was extremely humiliating. I needed the money that day, I needed every cent of it. I was counting on the money and I needed it that day. I wanted to borrow the car and I asked my mother for the car and she said she wouldn't give it to me, and I cursed at her. I had every right to curse at her. I was rip-roaring mad. I have every single right to curse at her—

Mother (*interrupting*): Before she went—

Julie (*shrieking*): That is none of her business. She is interrupting me, and it is none of her business where I go or where I have my hair done. It is my hair.

When Julie responds to her mother, the response is the complementary side of the mother's coin: she is petulant, demanding, and childish, and pretty soon mother and daughter are back on square one. The therapist is now in a position to request that Julie respond to her mother as an adult and negotiate from a position of mutual respect. This theme is played for thirty minutes, and whenever the dyad tries to change the theme, the therapist reframes it in terms of mutual respect. In order to resist the family pattern of cursorily dropping topics, he deliberately increases their duration or treats them as isomorphic—"You need to resolve it within a frame of mutual respect."

In the Poletti family Gina, a 14-year-old anorectic girl, vomits and takes laxatives to maintain herself at her pitiful weight. She was previously a "good daughter," and the parents feel helpless to deal with the strange behavior that the sickness imposes on their daughter. The family is composed of the father, 40; the mother, 30; Gina; John, her six-year-old brother; and the maternal grandmother.

The therapist moves the family away from the symptom and lengthens the transactions in which they talk about what they do to each other. His goal is to convey the message that the daughter's position is systemic and that she is caught in a conflict of loyalties between the mother, father, and grandmother. To transform the family diagnosis from "we are a helpful family trying to help a sick daughter who is possessed by a mysterious illness" to "we are all involved in a dysfunctional dance that is manifested most visibly in the daughter's symptom" is not a simple task. After thirty minutes into the first session, the therapist succeeds in eliciting from the mother a description of a conflictual transaction between herself and her daughter. This conflict offers the possibility of freeing the daughter from her triangulated position and thus becomes the frame for the therapist's interventions over the next hour. Keeping the family members involved in the nature of their conflictual transaction gives clarity and intensity to the therapeutic message.

Mother: When I dumped the garbage, there were two empty bottles of Ipecac after she had promised that she wouldn't take that for emetic purposes. I had some appetite depressant pills that had been prescribed for me by my doctor, and there were pills missing from the bottle. The salt shaker periodically disappears because she takes it in the bathroom and uses it to vomit with. She went through my drawers after I confiscated an infant syringe that I had to use to give herself enemas, and I found that hidden again in the bathroom.

Minuchin: What do you do when your lovely daughter does crazy things like that?

Mother: I—it makes me feel very angry, and then I try very hard to remember that she's sick and she's not really doing it to me on purpose, but then it makes me feel sad, so it's like going from anger to sadness.

Minuchin: You don't think she's doing that to you on purpose?

Mother: I think some of the things that she does, she does to manipulate me. I let her get away with a lot.

Minuchin (to Gina): Your mother says—and you know, it's a very interesting hypothesis—she says you do that on purpose to make her angry. Could that be true?

Gina: I don't do it on purpose.

Minuchin: Why does she think so? Talk with her—talk with her about her persistence that you are willfully doing certain things to get her mad. Talk with her about that.

The therapist moves the family's frame from their concentration on how to help a sick daughter to the question of how the daughter behaves and affects them. This issue has disappeared before the dramatic shadow cast by the serious symptom. For the next hour, the maintenance of this focus brings out hidden family dynamics.

Gina: Well, I didn't do it on purpose just to get you angry.

Minuchin (to mother): I want you to explore the way in which she does it against you, because I think that a lot of the things that she does are related to you.

The therapist maintains the focus. The mother then accommodates the therapist.

Mother: Ah—I'll tell you one thing that really bugs me is when I knock on your door and you're on the other side of the door and you purposely don't answer. I use the word "purposely" on purpose, because that's the message that I get.

Gina: Because I know that you are going to knock and open the door.

Mother: But I don't. I stand out there and I wait for you to answer the door.

Gina: Yeah, but when I go "what," you open the door. What good is that?

Mother: We knock on the door, Gina, and we ask if you are there, and when you don't answer, we knock a second time, and then we open the door. Do you know why?

Gina: Still, when I say "what," you open the door. I might be dressing or something. I like to have my privacy, you know.

Mother: The reason why we come in after we knock the second time—and I say "we" because Daddy does the same thing—is because one morning the window was open and you were gone.

Minuchin: Do not include your husband because he has his own voice.

Mother: Okay, that's the reason why I do it—and because a couple of weeks ago, you were talking about doing things to yourself—suicidal tendencies. I never know what to expect behind that closed door because I feel that you have manipulated me into a corner of fear, and I resent you for doing that, and I—I get the feeling that I am helpless, at times, that I'm at your mercy, and that's not right—not the way parents should be—mothers and daughters should be.

Minuchin (to mother): You are being very helpless, and you are giving Gina a lot of power that she doesn't know what to do with. Continue talking about the kind of things that she is doing to you that you don't like, that you find disrespectful, and that disturb you.

The therapist's intervention serves to ensure the continuity of the focus. He sees the mother's attempt to bring her husband into the transaction as one of the signals that the family members send when a transaction reaches a dangerous or stressful threshold, and thus he frames the father out, maintaining the mother and daughter in this transaction longer than is their habit.

Mother: One of the things that bothers me very much is the way in which you curse. I don't like that at all.

Gina: I get mad. Kids do it in school, so I get it from them.

Mother: I don't care whether they do it in school or not. I don't want you to do it at home.

Gina: And you do it, too, so why—

Mother: So what! I'm not 14 years old.

Gina: Well, you still do it.

Mother: That has nothing to do with what we are talking about. I don't like it when you do it at home; I don't like when you answer me back. Did you like it last night at the table when I hit you? Was that nice?

Gina: I don't care!

Mother: Well, I'm telling you that as long as you pursue a course of being disrespectful, that you're going to expect some kind of flack, because I'm not going to do that. It's fine for you to have privacy and rights of your own—I believe in that—but when you step on other people's rights and when you are disrespectful, then you'd better be tuned into the idea that there's going to be some flack because there will be.

Minuchin (to Gina): Can you defend yourself?

The therapist challenges the daughter to continue in the conflict.

Gina: Well, you don't have any respect for me. You expect me to have respect for you, but you don't have any for me.

Mother: That's not true. That's an absolute, outright lie.

Gina: Then why can you call me all those obscene names and everything, but I can't call you anything?

Mother: Because I'm not 14 and I'm your mother.

Gina: I don't see that that makes a difference.

Mother: You don't think that makes a difference? Then in other words, the message I'm getting from you is that you could really operate in this whole family structure without a mother. Is that right?

Gina: I didn't say that.

Mother: Well, if I'm just going to be something that can be answered back and something that can be cursed at and so what, etc., etc., the message I'm getting is that you could care less whether I'm here or not. And I have been vehemently screaming about the fact that I feel that you're trying to take my place in this family.

The continuing conflict shows the mother and daughter moving through a series of isomorphic themes locked in the same symmetrical transaction. The last statement, where the mother defines the daughter as being the challenger and the winner, shows the mother to be in a strange and powerless position. There has been a shift from the daughter as a victim of her illness to the daughter and mother as locked in a conflict for control. The therapist can posit, at this point, that the daughter is supported by the father or grandmother, or is in a coalition with both, against the mother. By maintaining the focus of the mother-daughter conflict beyond its usual threshold, the therapist highlights the position of the daughter as a puppet in the midst of a complex conflict.

Gina: I'm not trying to take your place.

Mother: Well, that's the feeling I get—like when I can't find anything because you go around and rearrange my kitchen.

Gina: Well, you never clean it, so I'm the only one that cleans it—

Mother: But that's not your business. The way in which I run the house—

Gina: Well, me and Nanny do it, too, so you can't always blame it on me.

Mother: And Nanny has her own place to take care of.

Gina: I know, but sometimes you put things away and you blame me for it.

Mother: I would prefer that both of you stay out.

Gina: Then it would look really sloppy.

Mother: Well, that's my—that's my affair, not yours. Just like it's my affair what I should be feeding your brother.

Minuchin (to father): Let me ask you, what do you do when two members of your family are having an argument?

Father: I am not sure—I am not sure what to do—

Minuchin: No, don't tell me. You intervene in that situation. Go ahead. Just do something.

The therapist maintains the same focus but expands the number of participants, asking the father to enact his part in the drama. The temptation is great to explore the depth of the mother-daughter dysfunctional relationship, but paradoxically, an exploration of this issue would decrease the affective intensity and bring the therapist in as a member of a triangle and a conflict diffuser. By maintaining himself as a time gatekeeper and introducing the father into the conflict, which now also includes Nanny, the therapist keeps the conflict alive.

Father (to wife): All right, I'll tell you. I can see Gina's point about calling her names and swearing. I can see that, and I'm just as guilty as you are, maybe more so.

The father takes Gina's position in the conflict.

Mother: Then how come you don't get the same kind of flack I do?

The wife extends the conflict to the spouse dyad.

Father: Ah—for some reason, and I don't—

Gina: Because you don't let me get your goat, that's why.

The daughter affiliates with the father.

Father: Well, I don't know. Maybe, I don't know, but that's not the point—

Mother: What about all the times before when your father was very quick with his hand? Who was the person who had the long fuse then?

The mother requests that Gina shift loyalties.

Gina: Well, sometimes you don't have short fuses.

The daughter accepts the mother's message.

Father: Yeah, but this doesn't alter the fact, you know, you're saying things about a sloppy house and everything else which are not true. Okay?

Gina: But—

Father: Your mother works all day long, and you can't expect her to come home and cook and clean and have everything nice and neat. There are many times when you have been asked to do something and you give us a big hassle about it. Yet when you feel like cleaning something up that Mommy doesn't necessarily want you to clean, you go ahead and do it anyway. I think this is the kind of thing that annoys her—and it annoys me.

The husband affiliates with the wife after the daughter shifts loyalties.

Minuchin (to grandmother): Mrs. Sansone, you have a certain wisdom because you are older. What do you think about the happenings in your family?

Grandmother: Um-hum. Well, I would say to Gina that she should try a little harder to show respect to her parents, because if I did what you are doing to your parents now, we would have got the back of the hand.

Gina: That was then. This is now.

Grandmother: No, honey, respect is respect, and you don't say it was then, or now, or tomorrow. If you want respect from your parents, you have to show them respect, too. *(To mother.)* Now that starts with you, Mara. All right? *(To therapist.)* Mara does bother me when she loses her temper, and a couple of times I said to her when she called Gina names, "Don't say that." Correct, Mara?

Mother: Um-hum.

Now all the participants have played their part in the family drama. The father enters into the conflict by first disqualifying his wife and then taking her side. The grandmother first challenges the granddaughter, but then sides with her and criticizes her own daughter's functioning as a mother. The therapist, by keeping himself out of the transactions, maintaining the focus, directing the entrance of the participants, and lengthening the time of their involvement, has increased the intensity of conflict in a family of conflict diffusers. Half an hour later, after several repetitions, Gina's position as the family weathervane has become clear.

Minuchin: So you are acting, really, in strange ways, Gina. You're acting as if you are six, and you're acting as if you are over 60, like your grandma. And both of your parents accept that, so it's not your fault. It's absolutely not your fault if you are running this household. But, Gina, you are caught because you are saying to your father the kinds of things that you think your mother wants to tell your dad, so you amplify Mother's voice. You are saying to your mommy the kind of things that you know your grandma and your father say to your mother. So you are just the voice of everybody in this family. You don't have your own voice. You are the puppet of the ventriloquist. Have you ever seen a ventriloquist? Sit on your mother's or your grandma's lap. Just for a moment, sit on her lap. (*Gina obeys.*) Now tell your mother the way in which she should change, thinking like grandmother.

Gina (using the disembodied voice of a ventriloquist's puppet): You should be a lot less sloppy.

Minuchin: Say to your mother the kind of things that your father wants to say.

Gina: Pick up your clothes off the floor.

Minuchin: Okay. It's extraordinary, Gina. You have developed into the ventriloquist's puppet in this family.

After the family presents their way of transacting, the therapist creates a dramatic scenario. He gives the family a powerful metaphor of the way in which they are interlocked—a way that is manifested openly in Gina's symptomatology.

CHANGING THE DISTANCE

Family members develop through life a sense of the "appropriate" distance to keep from each other. There is an apocryphal story about a meeting between two family therapists, Braulio Montalvo and Paul Watzlawick—in which Montalvo, who feels more comfortable when he is close to people, would take a step closer to Watzlawick who would withdraw two steps, to be followed by Montalvo's three steps forward, to be again followed by Watzlawick's retreat. By the end of their chat, they had gone around the room three times. Reportedly, their chat was about appropriate distances among people.

The movements back and forth that the two therapists did to maintain themselves "correctly" spaced were done automatically and out of awareness. The same experience can be undergone by the reader at any party where he gets closer to a person than feels appropriate to him.

This is true not only of measurable physical distance but also of less visible psychological distances. Changing the automatically maintained distance may produce a change in the degree of attention to the therapeutic message.

The utilization of the office space is a significant tool in the delivery of the therapeutic message. If the therapist talks with a small child, the child will listen and hear better if the therapist becomes shorter and physically closer, preferably touching the child. If the therapist wants to emphasize a serious message, he may get up, move toward a family member, stand up in front of him, and talk with the appropriate pitch and tempo, using silences for emphasis. He may do all that without being aware of his movements, just letting himself be directed by his sense of the need for intensity in the therapeutic message and his trust that the family members will direct his movement by their feedback.

The therapist can also increase intensity by changing the position of the family members vis-à-vis each other, making them sit together to highlight the significance of their dyad or separating a member to intensify his peripherality. In the Hanson family, the therapist asks the son to sit near his father, recreating the situation of overprotective enmeshment that characterizes their dyad, and then delivers his message about autonomy while getting physically closer to them.

RESISTING THE FAMILY PULL

Sometimes "not doing" can create intensity in therapy. This is especially true when the therapist does not do what the family system "wants him to do." Therapists are necessarily and unwittingly inducted into the family system as members of the therapeutic system. Sometimes this induction serves to maintain dysfunctional family homeostasis. By resisting the system's induction, a therapist brings intensity into therapy.

Some of the techniques used by Carl Whitaker as an unmovable therapist are in this vein, as is his concern at the beginning of therapy about winning the battle for leadership. This battle can start even before he has seen the family, in the discussion over the telephone about the number of participants in the session. Although instances of not being pulled by the family system are sometimes heroic or dramatic, they are also frequently of the most undramatic nature, since the resistance of the therapist to this pull is continuous throughout therapy.

For instance, the Williams couple were in therapy for two months, during which time they made considerable progress in dealing with their difficulties. They were able, in fact, to get beyond the point where in the past they usually diffused their difficulties by involving a third person, and could now bring some of their disputes to the point of resolution.

Then one week the wife calls the therapist and says she would like to speak to him alone at the beginning of the next session, and the therapist agrees. The wife and therapist retire to his office at the start of the session while the husband waits in the lobby.

Wife: Frank doesn't understand me. Every time I mention my concerns about my mother, he gets mad.

Fishman: This is between you and Frank. He needs to be here to respond.

The goal is to strengthen the relationship between the spouses. To allow the wife to complain about her husband to the therapist would not only involve the therapist inappropriately in their marriage but would also lose an opportunity for the husband and wife to resolve their differences themselves. By refusing to listen to the wife about the husband, the therapist gives intensity to the therapeutic message that the couple's transactions are complementary.

The Genet family consists of the mother, an artist in her mid-thirties, and three children, ages 15, 14, and 12. The husband left two years ago, and since then, life has been extremely chaotic for the family. The children stay out to all hours and attend school sporadically; the dishes pile up, with no fixed duties or rules for anyone.

The mother, a young-looking woman dressed in jeans and a tee shirt which says "Grateful Dead," sits slouched in her chair like the children. In fact, one has to do a double take to ascertain that she is not just one of the kids. The therapist sees that this is a "left-bank" family in which the mother, who has a Bohemian life style herself, is very uncomfortable setting rules for her kids. The therapeutic goal is to help to create a generational boundary in this family so that there is an executive subsystem.

Throughout the course of therapy the children and especially the mother invite the therapist to intervene and set limits. The pressure is tremendous for the therapist to activate and "help this family into shape." The therapeutic goal remains, however, to get the mother to assume the role of the leader for her family. For the therapist to assume this job would only allow the mother to continue as a helpless person. The correct intervention for the therapist in this situation consists of resisting the induction into the role of "helper" for the family. Otherwise, he will only contribute to the mother's displacement from an executive role.

Enactment is like a conversation, in which therapist and family try to make each other see the world as they see it. Intensity can be likened to a shouting match between the therapist and a hard-of-hearing family. Therapeutic efficiency can be drastically undercut by a therapeutic orientation that lets a therapist assume a correct message has been heard just because it has been sent, and by the rules of etiquette that incline people to fake understanding rather than appear rude. The family must truly hear the therapist's message. If they are hard of hearing the therapist will have to shout.

10 Restructuring

The therapist presses a diabetic girl's wrist. "Do you feel this?" he asks the parents.

"Yes, I do," the father says, indicating his own wrist. "Here. It feels like pins and needles."

"I have very poor circulation today," the mother says, apologizing for not sharing the experience.

In another family, the mother of a hospitalized 19-year-old anorectic insists on going to the hospital because she feels that her daughter is upset. When she arrives at the hospital, her daughter confirms her perception. In a session conducted later, the identified patient, her two adolescent sisters, and the father assure the therapist that the mother "knows" if any of them are in difficulty.

Neither of these families is prone to mystical experiences. Nor are the experiences themselves mystifying. The experience of belonging is characteristic of all family transactions. But the members of these families belong too well. Functioning as individual wholes has been subordinated to belonging.

The weakness of this type of family organization is that family members have difficulty evolving as differentiated holons. When they must function as autonomous entities, they may face a serious crisis. When the children reach late adolescence and must begin to separate from the family, psychotic breaks and psychosomatic illnesses can occur.

A therapist working with such families will have to interfere with their overly harmonious interactions, differentiating and delineating the boundaries of the family holons to make room for flexibility and growth. Functional families are complex systems, "made up of a large number of parts that interact in a non-simple way." These parts, or family holons, are interrelated in a hierarchical order. And as in all complex systems, the "intracomponent linkages are ... stronger than intercomponent linkages."[1] That is, transactions among members of a holon are stronger than the transactions that connect holons. The holon is therefore a highly significant context for its members.

Individuals belong to a multiplicity of holons, fulfilling different roles in each. In each holon, segments of their experiential repertory are activated. The skills appropriate in one holon may or may not be elicited in others, but they all become part of the possible repertory. Growing up in a functional family is a flexible process that results in a multifaceted individual who can adapt to changing contexts.

There is a built-in flexibility to a complex system, but there is also an enormous redundancy. "All human activity," Peter Berger and Thomas Luckmann remark, "is subject to habitualization. Any action that is repeated frequently becomes cast into a pattern, which can then be reproduced with an economy of effort and which, *ipso facto,* is apprehended by its performer as that pattern ... 'There we go again' now becomes 'this is how these things are done.' " Without a firm sense that this is how things are done, the individual cannot have the security to explore and grow. But the danger in the situation is that "There is a tendency to go on as before ... This means that institutions may persist even when ... they have lost their original functionality or practicality. One does certain things not because they *work,* but because they *are* right."[2]

Therapy is a process of challenging "how things are done." A major target of the challenge is the family subsystems, as these are the context for the development of complexity and competence.

Because therapy entails a challenge to family structure, the therapist must understand the normal development of families and the pervasive power that the rules of holons have in the development of family members. The nature of this development is seen in an interview conducted by Patricia and Salvador Minuchin as part of a research project on normal families.

The Tashjian family includes a couple in their late twenties with one child, a very active and competent two-year-old named Frank. The interview is conducted in such a way as to elicit parental controlling responses.

At one point, when the child moves across the room and spills pieces of chalk that are in a box, we ask the parents to have Frank put the spilled chalk back inside the box. The father, who has been talking to us with his back to the boy, turns around toward the child and in a peremptory tone of voice says to him, "Frank, put the chalk in the box," then turns back and continues talking to us. The boy puts one chalk in the box and then continues running around the room. The mother gets up, stands near the box, and says in a firm but friendly tone of voice, "Frank, come here and put the chalk in the box." Frank comes to where she is standing, begins to pick up the chalk, then after a while gets up without finishing the task and goes to another corner of the room. The mother kneels down near the box and asks Frank to come back, saying, "Finish picking up the chalk." At this point, the father turns in his chair and, in the same peremptory tone of voice, says, "Frank, put the chalk in the box," then turns around again and continues talking with us. The child moves toward where the mother is kneeling and begins to finish the operation, at which point the mother returns to her chair. The child leaves one piece of chalk on the floor and moves away, whereupon the mother says something along the lines of, "Go finish, Frank. If not, I will get up," and the child finishes the operation. This is a simplified description of a very complicated operation among three people. What is interesting is that when the parents afterward describe the process, both the mother and father identify the father as the person who is competent in controlling Frank and the mother as soft and inefficient. Yet observation shows that the parents in fact have two different styles of implementing control and that, in some way or other, their styles tend to be complementary. Although the father adds vocal intensity whenever he feels that the mother needs his help, the mother is clearly efficient in her own style and indeed most of the implementation of control is done by her. The question, therefore, is why the parents are unable to observe the data that are so evident to us as interviewers. Since the mother is efficient and competent in the area of control, how is it that everyone in the family agrees that she is inefficient in this area? Undoubtedly the mother's efficiency and competence are acknowledged in other areas in the family holon, as well as in extrafamilial groups. But in the parental holon, her framing as soft and inefficient is somehow necessary for its harmonious functioning. The data are therefore organized by the parents so that the stern voice of the father is given an added weight in effectiveness, which maintains the rules of the family organization.

This power of the context to organize the data and to maintain definitions of self and others is evident to everybody who has grown up in a family. In the Minuchin family, the notion that I had ten thumbs was not dispelled, challenged, or changed by my expertise as a horseman, my competence in playing bocci, or my skill at car mechanics in my father's business. These competencies were defined rather as part of my acknowledged responsibilities in the family, or as belonging to the extrafamilial, and my image as a child with ten thumbs remained intact within the context of the family. As a matter of fact, I protected this image, as when I learned how to swim without letting my parents know, and maintained that secret from them for three years, long after I was already an expert swimmer, because my mother was afraid that I would not be able to learn and would drown.

The daily transactions in a subsystem tend to organize the data of living together in ways that maintain the nature of the relationship unchallenged for as along as possible. In my case, the homeostatic laws clearly worked; and my dexterity and competence in handling things developed and were framed in transactions with my father and in the extrafamilial, which allowed the protective relationship between my mother and myself to be maintained. In effect, my ten thumbs and her nurturance were a behavioral unit. It is interesting that my sense of self as a ten-thumbed person remained intact, while my sense of self as a competent individual developed equally strongly in other areas; they grew up side by side in different holons. Only when, after marriage, I made some furniture that we needed and got the support and encouragement of my wife, was it possible for me to introduce all my learned competence in the extrafamilial into the interfamilial. This new definition of self became supported and expanded in my relationship with my spouse.

Murray Bowen, impressed by the power of these subsystems to remain symbolically effective even though people have left home, suggests that one way of challenging these definitions is to "go back" to the family of origin and change the nature of the transaction, not in the past, but in the present.[3] A more direct way of intervention is to facilitate in the therapeutic system the appearance of functions that family members carry in one holon and generalize them into others. There are three major techniques that challenge the holon structure of the family. The techniques of boundary making are designed to change the participation of members of different holons. Unbalancing changes the hierarchy of people within a holon. And complementarity challenges the concept of a linear hierarchy.

11 Boundaries

Boundary making techniques regulate the permeability of boundaries separating holons. The governing concept is the observation that participation in the specific context of a specific holon requires context-specific responses. People are always functioning with only part of their repertory. Potential alternatives can be actualized if the individual begins to act in another subsystem, or if the nature of his participation in a subsystem changes. Boundary making techniques can be aimed at the psychological distance between family members and at the duration of interaction within a significant holon.

PSYCHOLOGICAL DISTANCE

Often the way family members sit in a session indicates family members' affiliations. This is a soft indicator, which the therapist should accept only as a first impression that must be investigated, corroborated, or dismissed. The therapist will monitor spatial indicators, and also a variety of others. When a family member is talking, the therapist notices who interrupts or completes information, who supplies confirmation, and who gives help. These are, again, soft data, but they give the therapist a tentative map of who is close to whom, what the affiliations, coalitions, and overinvolved dyads or triads are in this family, and what patterns express and support the structure. He can then use either cognitive constructs or concrete maneuvers to create new boundaries.

The therapist with the Hanson family uses a cognitive construct to

146

delineate a boundary between two people. Five minutes into the session, he asks Alan, "Do you know Kathy's boy friend?" and Kathy answers. A moment later he asks Alan how old Dick is, and Kathy answers a split second ahead of Alan. The therapist now has two instances of the same type of intrusion, and he says to Kathy, "You're helpful, aren't you? You take his memory."

Phrases like these are cognitive indicators that separation is desirable. Experienced therapists collect a number of them that catch their imagination and become spontaneous responses in appropriate situations: "You take his voice." "If she answers for you, you don't have to talk." "You are the ventriloquist and she is the puppet." "Your hallucinated voices are not even yours; your father's voice is talking inside of you." "If your father does things for you, you will always have ten thumbs." "If your parents know when you need insulin, then you don't own your own body." These are idiosyncratic phrases of Minuchin's, who likes concrete metaphors. If a therapist borrows them, he must make them personal or, better, select his own phrases to highlight intrusion into psychological space, indicating and separating overinvolved dyads.

The therapist will be concerned with delineating boundaries among three people if dysfunctional dyadic transactions are maintained by the entrance of a third person as detourer, ally, or judge. In such cases the therapist may decide to maintain the separation of the overinvolved dyad as a way of helping them find alternatives to their conflict within their own subsystem. Or he may increase the distance between them by using the third person as a boundary maker, or by creating other subsystems that separate the overinvolved members. A common pattern is a disobedient child, an incompetent mother, and an authoritarian father. Their dance is a variation of the theme: child disobeys, mother overcontrols or undercontrols, child again disobeys, father enters with a stern voice or a grim look, and child obeys. The mother remains incompetent, the child remains disobedient, and the father remains authoritarian.

Another variation of the same dance is that of the parents who have conflicts, expressed or implicit, which are not resolved. When increased stress in the spouse dyad activates the unresolved conflicts, the child misbehaves, or takes sides with the mother against the authoritarian father, or joins with the father against the incompetent and unfair mother, or becomes the helper, or the judge, of both parents. If, as in the Kuehn family, the therapist decides to focus on the mother-child dyad and to do so requires that he immobilize the husband, he may say to the husband,

"Since the mother and child are usually together when you are at work, it would be nice for you to join with me in observing how they resolve it," or, "Since the mother and daughter are both women and neither you nor I has had experience in being a four- or 27-year-old female, the mother must understand your daughter better. Let's observe their dance and see what we can learn."

Or the therapist may decide in this situation to expand the definition of the problem from the mother-child overinvolvement by introducing the father's participation in maintaining the child's symptomatology. In this strategy, he will keep the focus on the child but increase the father's participation in the parental subsystem so as to separate the overinvolved dyad. He might say to the parents, "When a four-year-old is taller than her mother, maybe she is sitting on the shoulders of her father," or, "A four-year-old is no match for her parents if they pull together," or, "If you cannot handle a young kid, maybe you are pulling in different directions," or, "You two must be doing something wrong. I don't know what it could be, but I am sure if you think together, you will find out what it is, and moreover, you will find out the solution," or, "As things go, you are defeating each other, and in some way you are hurting and exploiting a child that both of you love very much, so we will need to find a way in which you help each other so you can help your child." This support of the parental subsystem aims at increasing both the psychological distance between the mother and child and the proximity between the spouses, giving them a common task as parents.

If the therapist decides to concentrate on the spouse dyad and their dysfunctional transaction and in that way to separate the overinvolved mother-child dyad, he will have to handicap the child's detouring strategy. He may say to the child, "You are a nice, protective, and obedient child by misbehaving . . . having a headache . . . failing in school, whenever your parents feel uncomfortable with each other," or, "When you explain your parents' behavior, or when you support your mother or father, I am fascinated by how fast you move from being ten years old to being 65 or 208 years old, and then running back to become four years old. But isn't it strange when you become your mother or father's grandmother? I will help you grow down. Bring your chair near me and be quiet while your parents deal with issues that concern them, where you don't have any reason to be, and no competence whatsoever." Or the therapist can tell one or both of the parents, "I want you to help your child to grow down by asking her to be quiet while you two discuss your issues."

Boundaries between subsystems are also necessary, and if parents intrude in sibling conflicts, or adolescents disqualify parents or intrude
into the spouses' area, or grandparents join with grandchildren against
their parents, or spouses bring their parents into coalition against their
spouses, the therapist has available a variety of boundary making techniques. Sometimes the therapist introduces a rule at the beginning of
therapy. He may say: "In this room, I have only one rule. It is a small
rule, but apparently very difficult for this family to follow. It is that no
person should talk for another person, or tell another person how this
person feels or thinks. People should tell their own story and own their
own memory." Variations on this rule allow the therapist to enforce
boundaries and to punctuate family members' intrusion into other members' psychological space as "disobedience to the rule." Intrusions, affiliations, or coalitions can be blocked as talking for another person, or
imagining that person's thoughts and future actions.

The therapist may create subsystems with different tasks. For instance, if children are involved in an argument, the therapist may invite
the interfering parents to join the therapist in an observing, "adult"
group "because children think differently these days than in our time
and may have solutions that we couldn't even imagine." Or he may ask
the parents to give the children the task of resolving a problem and, once
they have reached a solution, to talk it over with the children, supporting in this manner the executive function of parents but also ensuring
their nonintrusiveness. Or the therapist may ask one spouse to help the
other not to intrude into the children's arguments by squeezing the hand
of that spouse when he intrudes, while suggesting that they also pay
close attention to the children's communication, so that after they have
finished, the parents can comment from a parental point of view. Or he
may suggest that the parents and children separately and simultaneously discuss a family issue from their different points of view and that,
after they have finished, each group will tell the other how they see it,
thereby creating two subsystems that can function simultaneously without interfering with each other. The therapist may join as an observer,
or as a participant in one of the groups, or may move from one to the
other. Or the therapist may tell a grandparent that, since he has the
wisdom of age, the therapist is interested in hearing his observations
after he has carefully listened, without interfering, to the discussion between parents and children.

The therapist can also use concrete spatial maneuvers to change the
proximity between family members. Movements in space are universally

recognized as representative of psychological events or emotional transactions among people. Family members of different socioeconomic groups, adults and even young children recognize the metaphors of spatial closeness or distance as expressions of emotional connectedness. Changing the spatial relationships of family members in the session is a boundary making technique that has the advantages of being nonverbal, clear, and intense. The "world stops" when family members stop whatever they are doing and change positions with one another. This intervention has the added advantage of high visibility for family members who are not involved in the transaction. It has become almost a trademark of Minuchin to move people about in a session and to change places myself as a way of expressing changes in my emotional connectedness with family members.

The therapist may conduct himself as a spatial boundary maker, using his arms or body to interrupt eye contact in an overinvolved dyad. This maneuver can be accompanied by a change in the position of chairs so as to handicap the sending of signals, and it may be further reinforced by a statement like, "You are talking to your brother; you don't need your father's help," or, "Since you know this event better because you were there, consult your memory instead of using your mother's."

The therapist may request family members to change chairs in order to signal his support of a subsystem. For example, if the husband and wife sit separated by a child, he may say to the child that she should exchange seats with one of her parents so that they can talk directly instead of across her. If the therapist makes his directive clear and logical, family members usually comply. The therapist may get up and decrease his distance from the person of whom he requests the change if he thinks that this is necessary. This change in proximity between the therapist and the family members makes resistance more difficult.

In therapy, these techniques are not clearly separated; generally, in fact, they mix with and reinforce each other. The Smith family with a psychosomatic child is a case in point.

> *Therapist:* Mr. Karig, you seem to have a difference of opinion with your wife about that. Speak with her about your differences of opinion. (*General laughter from all four teenage children and the parents.*)
>
> *Father:* That's funny, because we never talk to each other.
>
> (1) *Therapist:* Well, you need to now, to resolve this difference between you.

Father (*to therapist*): I believe that Jerry—(*Therapist indicates that husband should talk to wife. Husband glances at his spouse and continues talking to the therapist. Several children begin making noises.*)

(2)

Therapist: No, speak to your wife. We will all listen, but you must speak with your wife. (*Makes a gesture that divides the parents from both himself and the rest of the family.*)

(3,4,5)

Father (*to therapist*): I know it's important, but it seems—

Therapist: No. Here, turn your chair a little so it's easier to see her. (*Helps husband turn his chair.*) And you, too, Mrs. Karig. (*Rotates her chair so she faces her husband. At this point the therapist turns his head and looks out the window. All the children remain silent.*)

(6,7)

(8)

Father (*turning and addressing his wife*): It seems like every time we start talking we end up saying things—

Mother (*to husband*): Who is usually right? Just answer me that.

This sequence, which takes about thirty seconds, contains at least eight boundary-making operations. The therapist verbally delineates the husband-wife subsystem (1), reinforces it with a hand gesture (2), and repeats it verbally (3). The children are excluded with both a verbal suggestion and hand gestures (4,5). The parents are realigned spatially to face each other and put their backs to the children (6,7). Finally, the therapist withdraws his contact by averting his head (8), whereupon the couple begin an extended discussion without interruption. The boundary making is successful because the therapist uses a variety of maneuvers until the desired isolation of husband and wife is accomplished. If one of the children persists in interrupting, the therapist may use his body to block the interruption, or move the child's chair farther away from the parents, or ask her to turn her chair to face another sibling, or tell the parents, "Invite one of your children to comment only when both of you agree to allow this." If the parents comply, then the therapist is no longer needed as a boundary maker. They will be doing it themselves.

Boundary making in this session, though conceptually simple, is very difficult for the therapist because he feels pressure from both spouses to join their subsystem. After he has asked the husband and wife to talk together, they continue talking to the therapist. If he responds to them, he will support the dysfunctional transaction that always includes another member to avoid conflict. In fact, he will undo what he is seeking to accomplish. The therapist in this segment avoids eye contact by looking out the window. For a therapist who in similar situations does not have a window available, concentration on a favorite toe would serve equally well, or take notes or doodle.

In the Brown family, the boundary making occurs around the father-daughter dyad. The family is seeking help for their 14-year-old daughter, Bonnie, who has been referred for intractable asthma. Her sisters, aged 18 and 17, are present in the session. Bonnie and her father begin a conversation about her school work. Halfway through the first exchange, their conversation activates the other family members. One sister says pertly that Bonnie should not have taken math. The mother assails the father for not helping Bonnie with her work. The other sister starts talking about her own school work.

The therapist, Ronald Liebman, moves Bonnie's chair so that she is facing her father and tells the father and daughter to continue their conversation. When the oldest sister tries to intervene, the therapist says to Bonnie, "This is between you and your father. Whenever you try to make your voice heard, your helpful family shuts you up with their helpfulness. Don't let them do that to you." The father and daughter continue, and shortly afterward the mother begins to speak. Liebman holds his hand up, signaling that the conversation is between Bonnie and her father. The next time someone interrupts, Bonnie herself says, "Wait a minute, please." The boundary making is now maintained by a family member.

In drawing a boundary around the father-daughter dyad, the therapist first uses a spatial arrangement. He moves Bonnie's chair, demarcating a subsystem: father and youngest daughter. This makes talking easier for the two and harder for those who would interrupt. Then he instructs Bonnie to delineate a boundary around her conversation. Later, he signals the others to stay out.

He could have done this in other ways. He could have asked the father to keep the others out, or he could have kept them out himself, or both. These would be essentially isomorphic interventions, and the reasons that the therapist selects one and not the others are idiosyncratic to the particular therapist in a particular context. The therapist also effectively uses his presence to etch boundaries by selectively directing his attention to the conversation between father and daughter. When others speak, he pays no attention. He gives cognitive corollaries to his interventions by calling to the attention of Bonnie and all other family members the incapacitating effects that their help has on Bonnie.

With the Brown family, the therapist uses a number of techniques for boundary making: rearrangement of physical space to indicate subsystems, utilization of himself to protect the subsystem from the intrusion of other family subsystems, and a reason for his support of the subsystem. The first two interventions are concrete maneuvers, the last a cognitive construct. In this situation they are sufficient to activate a family member, Bonnie, to protect the father-daughter subsystem. In the therapeutic process, a number of different boundary making techniques will need to be employed and used repeatedly before they can achieve sufficient intensity to produce structural change.

At times, the utilization of spatial metaphors may take the form of the rearrangement of chairs in two circles to protect two subsystems simultaneously, or the turning of a chair 180° to isolate or protect a member, or the removal of an empty chair or an ashtray or a pocketbook from between spouses to indicate the need for proximity. The closeness of the therapist to a member, his kneeling or touching her, or his standing high above her are all indicators of connectedness that do not require verbal or cognitive qualifiers.

In situations in which the executive subsystem includes an incompetent member and an intrusive, helpful, and competent member, the therapist may ask the "competent one" to observe from beyond the one-way mirror how the "helpless" member handles things when she is without the "competent" help. Another nonverbal technique is simply to ask parents to bring to the session only certain members of the family and not others, indicating in that way a separation of subsystems. Or the therapist may indicate who is to participate in different sessions.

In certain families with a chaotic style of communication, where there is continual interruption or simultaneous talking, the therapist may find that the threshold of noise is above his capacity for comfortable communication. He can then use artificial devices, such as inventing a game in which people sit silently in a circle and only a dyad or a triad may go into the middle to communicate; or the therapist provides the participants with an object (hat, chalk, key) to indicate which family members have the right to talk. In addition, whenever the stress in a session increases beyond the therapist's capacity to be effective, a diminution in the number of participants immediately creates a different subsystem with different alternatives for the reduction of stress.

DURATION OF INTERACTION

Extending or lengthening a process, which is one way of increasing its intensity, may also be utilized to demarcate subsystems or to separate them. In these situations, the content of the transaction is less important than the fact that the transaction occurs.

In the Kuehn family, after the mother is able effectively to control her daughter, the therapist brings in puppets and encourages the mother and daughter to play. This process is kept up for over twenty minutes without any interruption by the therapist, except for the introduction after ten minutes of the father as a playmate. The therapist is concerned not with the content of the transaction but only with keeping first the mother-daughter holon and later the mother-father-daughter holon in a pleasurable situation long enough to establish a complementary counterpoint with the accustomed controlling mother-daughter subsystem.

The previous techniques occur within the therapeutic system in the therapist's presence. The therapist is involved in monitoring the boundaries, if he is not actually a boundary himself. But to be effective, therapy must be maintained outside of the session. When a therapist is concerned with maintaining a particular subsystem, he may give the family homework to support the processes initiated in the session. His "ghost" then carries the therapeutic task. Practicing unaccustomed transactions in a natural setting facilitates structural change.

Like techniques used within the session, interventions outside the session can affect affiliations in space or time. In the Pulaski family, a widowed mother is overinvolved with her hypochondriacal 18-year-old daughter. The therapist gives the mother a task: find something to do that involves only herself. The mother, who is somewhat overweight, informs the therapist at the next session that she has joined a diet group. The task in this situation is contentless; it is up to the mother to select what is appropriate within her own life context. A task to increase the proximity of spouses could be an assignment. Each is to relate for a week in a way that will give satisfaction to the other, but without telling the other what the plan is. In the next session, the spouses are asked to describe the changes in each other.

In other cases, the therapist will assign tasks in precise detail. For instance, in a family with an overinvolved mother-son dyad with a peripheral husband, the therapist may direct the father to help the boy with his homework, or control the boy when he misbehaves, or teach the boy how to play soccer or do carpentry, with the explanation that, "Since you are a man and your son will grow to be a man, you should discipline

... or teach ... or play with him for the next week." A task of this sort can be supported by a statement of concern for the mother, such as, "Since your wife has been working so hard with Billy, it is important that she should take a week or two of rest." The specification of a time limit gives the family the framework of transition and experimentation and facilitates their participation in the search for alternative solutions.

A different technique for creating boundaries in overinvolved dyads is the use of paradoxical tasks, in which the therapist suggests or directs an increase in the proximity of family members of an overinvolved dyad or subsystem. For instance, she may direct an overprotective mother to increase her attention to a child's minor needs, or instruct an overinvolved spouse to keep closer track of his spouse's whereabouts. The aim of this technique is to increase the conflict between participants, which will be followed by an increase in their distance.

Various techniques of boundary making are used with the Hanson family, after the therapist has asked Alan to talk to his father.

Alan: Would you give me a hand, Peg?

Peg: Tell Daddy that you want to make decisions by yourself. If you really want to do it.

Alan: Yeah, I would like to be more independent, but I guess it's a habit of letting people do things for me, and I've gotten into it.

Peg: And I guess it's going to be very hard for Daddy to stop. It will be hard for all of us, but especially Daddy, because he and Mommy tend more to be protective. And it's going to take a long time, and it's going to take a lot on your part, too, to make decisions and say, "Well, look, I don't want Peg to help." You can't be afraid to say it.

Alan: Yeah.

Minuchin: Peg, do you find yourself frequently in the job of being the helper?

Peg: Yes.

Minuchin: Who else is asking you for help?

Peg: Uh—my mother.

The therapist tries to utilize a sibling to separate Alan from his over-protective and handicapping father. The content of their discussion is one of separation and individuation, but the therapist notes that Peg herself seems extremely comfortable in the role of helper. He assumes that Peg may also participate with other family members in the maintenance of dysfunctional transactions. His exploration of this hunch brings forth the mother's utilization of Peg to maintain her own distance from her husband.

Minuchin: Pete, exchange seats with your mom, because I want your mother to talk with Peg. (*Pete unhooks his microphone to change chairs, and Peg starts to help him.*) No, let him do it. (*To Pete.*) Very good. You did it on your own. Nobody helped you. Maybe you will still be safe, Pete, since nobody will help you. Mom, talk with Peg because I think Peg gets herself saddled with helping a lot in the family.

Since the therapist, by this point in the session, has seen that three dyadic subsystems in the family operate with intrusive overprotection, he will automatically look at all transactions that occur in terms of their ability to support or curtail competence and autonomy. As a result, he supports Pete's autonomy by blocking the unnecessary help from Peg and by affiliating with him in his competence. Then the therapist moves back to the mother-daughter subsystem.

Mother: She does. Peg wants—
Minuchin: Talk with *her* about how you saddle her.
Mother: About how I saddle her with the problems?
Minuchin: Yeah.
Peg: Right. Well, I never realized it. It just happened that grandmother—
Mother: My mother used to live with us, and she was around all the time when Peg was growing up, and then when she wasn't there, I just automatically used to ask Peg—I didn't realize that I was putting pressure on Peg. I thought it was more or less conversation. Right, Peg?
Peg: Maybe you didn't realize it, but I knew that you wanted me to help you decide things.
Mother: I always considered it more like we would talk over things together and then I would make my own decision, but I think maybe you felt that it was left on your shoulders to make the decision.
Peg: A lot of times you did. You would say, "What do you think I should do?" or, "What do you think about this?" And I made a lot of decisions.

It becomes clear that the dyads—Kathy-Alan, Alan-father, Peg-Alan, Peg-mother, and mother-grandmother—all have a similar organization and that this is a family in which the enmeshment hampers differentiation. The therapist assumes that if Peg has replaced her grandmother in her relationship with her mother, she may be filling a vacuum in the mother's life created by a disengaged husband. The therapist goes on to investigate the functioning of the spouse subsystem.

Minuchin: You did ask Peg to make decisions?
Mother: Not about important things, like about if you're going to buy a house or something like that, but about—
Peg: About family things.
Mother: Yeah.
Minuchin: Family things. She would ask you?
Mother: Yes—I would ask her to help.
Minuchin: Father, where were you? You that are so helpful. You that are helping Alan. Where were you? Why didn't your wife ask you?
Father: I wasn't around too much then.
Minuchin: Oh, that's why. Are you saying that you were alone and that you used Peg because Nels was not around?
Mother: Nels was working two jobs for a long time. He's always working two jobs, but now he has more of an interest in the house. I feel Nels has time if it's something he's interested in, and if it's something he doesn't want to think about, he's just not there to hear it.
Minuchin: Peg, come here and move out from that center. Mom, you sit near your husband. You know, Peg, I think that it's a pity for you to be sitting here between them. I bet that you are too available. I bet you like that job.

The therapist changes the spatial arrangement of Peg, husband, and wife, separating the daughter from the spouse subsystem. He also gives a cognitive construct supporting his spatial metaphor. His strategy of working with dyads has elicited a picture of the mother-Peg subsystem as a structure inherited from the mother-grandmother subsystem. Both structures have kept the husband and wife at a comfortable distance from each other. The therapist continues activating the spouse subsystem.

Mother: How do you think we can go about correcting this mess?
Father: Well, I think I should start being home nights for one thing. I'll leave the other job—
Minuchin: Can you stop shaking your head, Peg? It's not your function.

The therapist blocks Peg from taking her habitual position as the third person in the spouse subsystem.

Father: Much as I feel I have to change an awful lot, I think you have to change.
Mother: In what way?
Father: Oh, general mannerisms, your attitude toward me personally. I feel very deeply hurt many times.
Mother: How?
Father: I feel you don't feel I am a full man—a full husband. I feel you look down on me many, many times.
Mother: How do I act that makes you feel I look down on you?
Father: Sometimes you don't have to act, you can just look.
Mother: But I don't understand what—like what do I do that gives you that impression? How do I—obviously I—
Father: I'm trying to look for an answer here.

The problem has now been transformed from a problem of a young man with severe psychological difficulties to a problem of a family with dysfunctional rules and subsystems that are not working as well as they might. As the problem has been transformed, so has the therapist's job. In the first part of the interview, it was indeed the therapist's job to spread the problem among family members, to reframe it so that what has been described as a problem of one becomes a problem of the family. Now the therapist must challenge the family organization that keeps the father peripheral. Unless the spouses are able to function well, independent of the children, Alan, Peg, Kathy, and Pete will have difficulty differentiating and separating from the family.

Father: You are not respectful of me.
Mother: I don't think I'm not respectful with you. I don't mean to be not respectful of you.
Minuchin: You said that she doesn't treat you as a full man. You make Nels feel that you are not on his side.
Mother: And I guess I have feelings that he doesn't understand me, either.
Father: I think we've been throwing this back at each other for a long, long time, and it's—
Minuchin: You have not been helpful. You, Peg, have not been helpful.

When the spouses get stuck in their blame-counterblame set, the therapist highlights Peg's triangulated position as a supporter of the husband-wife homeostasis and her lack of alternatives.

Peg: What do you mean? Now? Or in the past?

Minuchin: Whenever Mom chose to talk with you instead of talking with Dad. Will you resign from that job or are you stuck with it?

Peg: I don't know. Let me think for a minute. I don't think that my mother is going to stop—

Minuchin: Using you?

Peg: Yes, you're right.

Minuchin: It's a job that you like for life? Do you want that job for life?

Peg: No, because I'm not her mother. I'm only 21 years old. If I wanted to be the mother, I'd get married.

The therapeutic affiliation with Peg acts to separate the mother and Peg. Peg then requests age-appropriate autonomy.

Minuchin: She's not using you as a mother really. She uses you when she feels she does not know how to talk with your father. (*To parents.*) So Peg is in between both of you. Who is on the other side?

Father: Oh, Peg is there with her mother and the mother is with Peg.

Minuchin: What about the other ones?

Father: Pete is fairly independent. He'll speak his piece. And Kathy is— I'd say she'll look at both sides. Alan will form an opinion, I feel, but he will keep it inside him rather than take sides.

Minuchin: Do you think he is taking sides but he is keeping it silent?

Father: I feel so.

Minuchin: And with whom is he siding?

Father: I think Alan feels about his mother like I do. I honestly, sincerely feel that. I don't think he wants to take sides, but I feel Alan feels a lot of times I may be right, but he'll never say it.

The therapist's simple strategy of boundary making throughout this session highlights a dynamic of triangulation supporting severe pathology. The development of the spouse subsystem was handicapped in the beginning of the marriage by the mother's mother, who lived with the couple and joined in a coalition with her daughter against her husband. The children growing up in the family joined with the mother-grandmother subsystem, while the father chose life as a workaholic and also an alcoholic, which maintained him in the family as a disengaged member. Alan chose a coalition with the losing side. But the drama of choosing sides is played out daily in silence, in highly nonvisible transactions. Now that the therapist has a map, identifying the problem of the family and the goals of therapy, he can, with a measure of wisdom, lead the family out of its difficulties.

The techniques of boundary making are easily learned and can therefore be used effectively even by therapists who do not have theoretical structure to order and integrate the phenomena they observe or produce. But in such cases, boundary making, even when elegantly realized, remains an isolated phenomenon. The point of boundary making is not that it is possible, but that it is done for a reason. If the therapist knows where he is going, he will find the vehicle.

12 Unbalancing

In boundary making techniques the therapist aims at changing family subsystem membership, or at changing the distance between subsystems. In unbalancing, by contrast, the therapist's goal is to change the hierarchical relationship of the members of a subsystem.

When the therapist and the family members join a therapeutic system, they enter into an explicit contract that defines the therapist as the expert of the system and the leader of the therapeutic endeavor. Consequently, mere entrance into the therapeutic system changes the family power structure. Everybody takes one step down, as it were, allocating to the therapist the power necessary for the utilization of her expertise. This shift will not be challenged by the family members as long as the therapist respects the family's own power allocation.

The problem is that the therapist will have to use herself, as a member of the therapeutic system, to challenge and change the family power allocation. Family members expect the therapist to be "firm but fair." They expect her either to support everyone's point of view in a balancing act that leaves things unchanged or to "judge" who is right from the objective position of an outside expert. Instead, the therapist joins and supports one individual or one subsystem at the expense of the others. She affiliates with a family member low in the hierarchy, empowering him instead of undercutting him. She ignores the family switchboard. She joins a family member in a coalition that attacks another family member. These operations handicap the recognition of the signals by

161

which family members commonly indicate to each other the appropriateness of their interpersonal behavior. The family member who changes position in the family by affiliation with the therapist does not recognize, or does not respond to, the family signals. He operates in unaccustomed ways, daring to explore unfamiliar areas of personal and interpersonal functioning, highlighting possibilities that were previously unrecognized.

Unbalancing a system may produce significant changes when individual family members are able to experiment with expanded roles and functions in interpersonal contexts. These changes may produce new realities for the family members. Since the reality of the family members is a matter of perspective and punctuation, any change in the hierarchical position in the family produces a change in the perspective of family members in relation to what is permissible in the transactions among members. Alternatives within all subsystems may therefore be uncovered and become possible.

There are two major problems with unbalancing techniques. One problem is ethical. Unbalancing techniques are, by definition, unfair. Although the therapist, with a systemic epistemology, interprets family members' behavior as maintained by the system, she adopts a linear epistemology temporarily, supporting one member's point of view. The therapist must pay close attention to the effect of these techniques on family stress, particularly to the difficulties faced by a low-power family member who is suddenly affiliated with the therapist. If the therapist perceives that the maneuver has reached an unbearable threshold, she may rescind or postpone, join other family members for a while before continuing her strategy, or convey to family members not joined that she will attend to them next. The therapist may also convey the hope that there are possibilities for new solutions in the change of perspective that unbalancing achieves.

The other problem with unbalancing techniques is the personal demands made on the therapist. Although it is possible to unbalance a family system by using cognitive constructs that allow distance between the therapist and family members, for the most part unbalancing techniques require proximity, participation, and temporary commitment to one family subsystem at the expense of others. The therapist whose preferred style tends to be objective and detached finds that learning these techniques enlarges her therapeutic repertoire usefully, but she may also find it hard going. Stress in the therapist-supervisor subsystem may also arise.

Yet these techniques can be among the most valuable the therapist develops. Take the Windsor family, with an alcoholic father, a martyred, overintellectual wife who can neither live with her husband nor live without him, and a bright but over-responsible eight-year-old girl who is expected to judge which of her parents is in the right. When the family comes to therapy after the spouses have tried to separate and failed, the therapist affiliates with the man. This is extremely difficult, since his long history of alcoholism and drug addiction have defined him as the deviant, and this deviant position is accepted not only by the rest of the family members but also by the mental health system that has intervened for long periods in the life of the family. The therapist's support for the man who has been defined as deviant is challenged by all family members in some way and is even difficult for the therapist, who shares with her culture a sense that the addict is expressing irresponsibility in preferring the deviousness of alcohol to the commitment and responsibility of caring for his family. Nonetheless, the therapist supports the father's sparkling sense of humor and directs him to help his wife with her depression.

Another problem for the therapist is to maintain the affiliation with the man even though she empathizes with the woman's sense of hopelessness and is challenged by the man during therapy to continue affiliating with him through periods of intoxication and addiction. The benefits for the family of this unbalancing technique are the possibility of developing alternative ways of relating to each other. Family therapists believe that, given a change in circumstances, people—even people who have been defined as deviant for many years—can experiment with alternatives that are made available to them. Such alternatives include in this case not only a change in the behavior of the identified patient, the man, but also the appearance of new behavior in the wife and daughter that supports the changed behavior of the total family.

Unbalancing techniques fall into three categories, according to the demands that they put on the therapist's personal involvement. The therapist may affiliate with family members, may ignore family members, or may enter into a coalition with some family members against them.

AFFILIATION WITH FAMILY MEMBERS

Therapeutic joining is, in essence, a technique of affiliation. The therapist confirms people, emphasizes their strength, and thus becomes a significant source of self-esteem to them. By using herself to create a context of trust and hope, the therapist facilitates the exploration of and experimentation with alternatives. To unbalance, the therapist uses her affiliation with one family member to change his hierarchical position in the family system. The focus on one family member changes the position of all family members. Though it is possible to unbalance by affiliating with a dominant member of a group, this technique is used mostly to support a peripheral family member or one in a down position. Feeling the therapist's affiliation, that person begins to challenge his prescribed position in the system.

In the Blaise family, a 13-year-old girl with school avoidance problems, who is overinvolved with her mother, came to therapy with the goal of trying to get medical permission for home tutoring. The therapist supports the mother's concern for the daughter, highlights the mother's difficulties at work since she never knows whether her daughter has gone to school or not, shows concern for the mother's loss of salary when she cannot go to work owing to the daughter's staying home, and in general frames her support of the mother as a concern for her heavy burden: having a daughter who refuses to go to school. His intervention highlights for the mother her exploitation by the daughter; the mother rebels, demanding that the daughter go to school.

The Clark family, composed of a father, a depressed mother, and a 25-year-old son who lives at home, came to therapy because of the mother's depression following the death of her younger son two years previously at age 21. It is clear that the family has since been organized around the mother-younger son subsystem with a peripheral father. The therapist assumes that the mother's depression is related to her fear of her last son's moving out, leaving her alone with her husband. The therapist concentrates on supporting the young man's position as a healer in the system, a substitute for the dead brother who monitored the distance between the father and mother. He confirms the young man's accomplishments as a math teacher in high school, interested in curriculum development. The therapist suggests that since the son is concerned about the mother's depression, he should encourage his girl friend to become equally concerned, so that both of them can support the mother. But the therapist also points out how the family is constricting the son's life and how his healing functions are leaving the father's capacity for support and nurturance unutilized in the family. The therapist's support of the son leads to his moving out of the home and to a change in the relationship between the husband and wife.

The Vogt family, composed of a mother and father in their fifties and two adult children, came to treatment because the mother is "psychotic." Everybody else in the family is "okay" and carries a mantle of martydom for enduring the mother's craziness. The mother is a childish woman who has learned, through years of contact with hospitals and therapists, a lack of constraint that befits the crazy. But she is also a nice-looking person with excellent taste, bright and tender. The therapist affiliates with her, asking why her family demands so little from her. He listens to her, confirms her intelligence, and asks her to begin to cook for her husband. When she responds with childish nonsequiturs, the therapist does not accept them. He reframes her craziness as support of a family who would not know what to do if she changed. From the affiliative position, the therapist increases his demands that she change her position in the family.

The therapist can use affiliation with a dominant member as an unbalancing technique, which creates a runaway situation. The therapist intensifies the family member's habitual function. The therapist's goal is to cross the threshold of the permissible in a family and to elicit a challenging response in other family members. A number of paradoxical tasks have this effect.

An example of runaway unbalancing occurs with the Henry family, which consists of a 19-year-old son and his divorced mother. The two of them live alone and are extremely isolated and enmeshed. They came to therapy originally because the boy had a psychotic episode. Following hospitalization, the young man returned to college and did fairly well. In the present crisis, as the young man's social life is developing, his mother is becoming increasingly depressed. One day they call their therapist and the young man reports that he is suicidal. He says he is afraid he is going to "jump out the window." The therapist tells the mother that he sees the son's suicidal threat as extremely serious and it is her responsibility to keep her son from harming himself. He gives the mother the assignment of keeping an eye on her son so that he does not jump out the window. No matter where he goes, the mother is to watch him. They are to sleep in the same room, and the mother is to attend class with the young man. The mother consents, because she, too, feels the gravity of the son's threat and is impressed by the therapist's description of his suicidal behavior as her responsibility. So the mother and son spend more time together than they have for years. She sits in class and goes around campus with him.

As the young man is taking a sailing class, they call the therapist to ask whether the mother should also go out sailing with him. The therapist says that indeed she must, since he might do something suicidal like jump out of the boat. So the next day, a rainy Saturday, mother and son go out in the sailing dinghy. After a few days the young man calls up stating that he wants to be freed from having his mother go everywhere with him. The mother is similarly motivated. The therapist, however, tells the mother that she should not allow her son to go out alone until she is convinced that he is not suicidal. Mother and son fight more than they have in years. The mother investigates adult education. The young man spends a good deal of time on the phone. Finally, the mother gets her son to assure her that he is not suicidal. Relieved, both go back to their everyday lives, each irked with the other and more autonomous than they have ever been.

Unbalancing techniques that use affiliation may require a maintenance of this strategy for a number of sessions. Alternatively, the therapist may shift affiliation to a different member in the same session. A case in point is the Kuehn family in which four-year-old Patti acts as an uncontrollable monster, the mother as an ineffective person, and the father as an authoritarian. The therapist's goal is to test the flexibility of the functioning of the family members, to see if the mother can become more effective and the father can develop a more nurturant and flexible attitude toward both mother and children. In the first half hour of the previously described session, the therapist supported the mother as a way of helping her to explore and actualize her capacity to function more effectively. Here, the therapist moves toward supporting the father, which requires an unbalancing of the system. The therapist's strategy is to underline and support the elements of the father's functioning that are positive and effective.

Minuchin (to father): Why does your wife think you are such a tough person? She feels that you are very tough, and she needs to be flexible because you are so rigid. I don't see you at all as a rigid person. I see you actually as quite flexible. How is it that your wife feels that you are rigid and nonunderstanding?

Father: I don't know. Lots of times I lose my temper, and that's probably why.

Minuchin: I have seen you playing with your daughters here, and I think you are soft and flexible and that you were playing in a rather nice and accepting way. You had initiative in your play; you were not authoritarian.

Father: Great self-image. (*Laughs.*)

Mother: Yeah.

Minuchin: That's true. That is what I saw. So why is it she sees you only as rigid and authoritarian and she needs to defend the little girls from you? I don't see you that way at all.

Father: I don't know. As I said, the only thing I can think of was that I lose my temper with them.

Mother: Yeah, he does have a short fuse.

Minuchin: Okay, but that doesn't mean that you are authoritarian and that doesn't mean that you are not understanding. Your play with your daughter here was filled with warmth; she enjoyed the way in which you play. So, some way or other, your wife has a strange image of you and your ability to understand and be flexible. Can you talk with her? How is it that she needs to be protective of your daughter from your short fuse?

The therapist's intervention is more of an affiliation with the father than a coalition against the mother. The therapist emphasizes the aspects of the father that are soft and nurturant. He emphasizes his flexibility and playfulness. All these characteristics of the father are inhibited in the family program, where he is accepted in his function as an authoritarian. The therapist's concern with the father is itself soft, playful, and nurturant, so that there is an enactment in the transaction between them of a forbidden element in the family organization, of the possibility that men can be nurturant and act tenderly. In response to this therapeutic intervention, the father becomes firmer in his request for change from the mother.

Minuchin: Talk with her about that because I think she is wrong.

Mother: That's basically what it is. I'm afraid of you really losing your temper, because I know how bad it is. They are little, and if you really hit them with a temper, you know, you could really hurt them, and you wouldn't want that, so that's why I go the other way to show them that everybody in the house doesn't have that short fuse.

Father: Yeah, but when you do that, that just makes it a little worse, because that makes Patti think that she's got somebody backing her. Do you know what I mean?

Mother: Um-hum. Yeah.

Minuchin: This is very clever and is absolutely correct, and I think that you should say it again because your wife doesn't understand that point.

Mother: No, I understand it.

Minuchin: No, I don't think you do. Say it to her again so that she hears it.

Mother: That I'm backing Patti up against you?

Father: And that's probably why she doesn't listen to you, because she looks at you as more of a playmate than as her mother. Someone she can run to.

Mother: Um-hum. I never realized—well, I guess—I guess I could see how she would. Yeah. But it's not my nature to be the other way.

Father: Well, maybe you can change your nature then.

Mother: Yeah.

The therapist continues his support of the father's unused functions in the family, emphasizing what is not acknowledged: the father's clarity of expression and his ability to understand both young children and transactional processes. In the extent to which the affiliation of the therapist with the father creates a distance between husband and wife, the husband becomes able to respond to his wife in a different modality. The man who has been characterized as the brute and the policeman in the family now approaches wife as a person of insight. The therapist supports the husband's challenge to the wife but does not himself challenge her.

Minuchin: Mr. Kuehn, why is your wife afraid of your temper?

Father: I don't know, to tell you the truth, because I don't think I ever did anything to her—

Mother: I've seen his temper.

Minuchin: Mr. Kuehn, when was the last time you beat your wife?

Father: I never beat my wife. I just threaten her. (*Laughs.*)

Mother: No, I'm really proud of that.

Minuchin: She talks as if you beat her regularly. (*Father laughs.*)

Mother: No, it's just a fear that I have. I've seen the temper, and he's completely out of control and it takes over.

Minuchin: Mr. Kuehn, when you have this temper, what things in your house have you destroyed? Dishes?

Father: No.

Minuchin: Furniture? Windows?

Father: No, I think the worst thing I did was hit a wall one time, that's all.

Mother: You put your fist through the wall one time, and a shoe another time.
Father: Yeah, I threw a shoe and hit the—
Minuchin: To whom do you throw a shoe?
Mother: At the wall.
Father: I threw it just one time.
Minuchin: And when you hit with your fist against the wall, did you really put your fist through the wall?
Mother: Not all the way through.
Father: Just a dent in it, that's all.
Mother: A dent in the wallboard.
Minuchin: The extent of your anger is that you discharge it within your area without destroying anything.

The therapist's support of the husband and the subsequent unbalancing of the system when the husband demands a change in the wife deactivates the family blueprint. The family reality then reappears: the father is the stern family disciplinarian, and the characteristics of flexibility, playfulness, and clear thinking that appeared in the previous segment are all erased by the irrational aspects of his way of functioning when he is "his true self." The therapist's challenge to this presentation of the husband takes the form of a concrete exploration of the "facts." The family has an accepted but unexplored myth of the father's destructiveness. The therapist opens up the myth for exploration. In the historical review of the facts in the therapist's presence, the family "truth" falls apart, and the therapist's affiliation with the father allows a different myth to emerge.

Father: Yeah, well, there is a reason for that though. When I was a kid, my father used to tear the house apart and—
Mother: Furniture and everything—
Father: —that's one thing I would never do. I've seen it happen.
Minuchin: That means that what your wife is afraid of is something that literally does not exist.
Father: Yeah, I guess so. Because, I don't know, those instances were years ago anyway, the few times I did that.
Mother: Yeah, but they're still locked in your memory, and you know—
Minuchin: No, no, no! You are not saying what is in *his* memory. What you are saying is that they are locked in *your* memory.

Mother: Right, and that's why I'm still afraid of him, because I know how out of control he can get.

Minuchin: Mr. Kuehn, she's selling you a bag of—of lies! Please do not buy it. She's selling you the idea of your temper, of your rigidity, of your destructiveness. But what I hear is that the most you have done is (*hits the chair*) that, maybe stronger.

Father: A lot strong—

Minuchin: How did you do it? Like that? (*Takes his shoe and slams it on the floor.*)

Father: That's right. (*Laughs.*)

Minuchin: And you did not hit anyone.

Father: Just the wall, yeah.

Minuchin: Okay, so what is she talking about? What is she selling?

Mother: Well, that scares me, that's enough to scare me.

Minuchin: What is she selling? She's selling an image of a monster, of somebody that one needs to be afraid of. I don't understand why you accept that your wife should think that you can hurt your little daughters when you are such a teddy bear.

Mr. and Mrs. Kuehn were childhood sweethearts. Mr. Kuehn's father was the town drunk, and he grew up with a fear of destructiveness and of the aggressiveness of his father toward his own mother and himself. Mrs. Kuehn, on the contrary, grew up in a family with a very controlling mother with whom she is still in almost daily contact and who emphasizes and supports her incompetence. When the Kuehns married, out of the weave of their individual lives they constructed a family myth of the father's destructiveness, which serves to program their individual functions in the family and a number of their transactions. The transactional patterns of avoidance between the husband and wife support the myth, which in return programs the patterns of avoidance. The wife, the husband, and the daughter have all agreed on the destructive aspects of the husband. The therapist's support of the husband is a challenge to this family truth. The therapist takes off his shoe and throws it on the floor, parodying the destructiveness. The husband is called a teddy bear, soft, and nurturant. The therapist relates to his softness at the time that the family is talking about his destructiveness. This is a challenge to the narrowness by which the family has programed the man's presentation of self in the family.

The change in context of the man in the therapeutic system puts him in a bind. To maintain the affiliation with the supporting therapist, he must change his old pattern of avoidance with his wife and actively challenge her to change in relationship to him and in relation to the daughter.

Minuchin: So I think this idea that you have, that your wife backs Patti to protect her from your temper, is something that you need to look at carefully. I think you are right—this is the way in which little Patti becomes a monster.

Father: That's funny, that's what I call her—the monster.

Mother: That's what he calls her—the monster.

Minuchin: But this is a monster of your creation. You are creating a monster.

Mother: Um-hum.

Minuchin: In a very lovely, bright, four-year-old, you are creating a monster, and that's unfair. I think it's unfair for parents to create a monster.

Father: It's unfair to the kid, too.

Minuchin (to wife): You need to change.

Mother: Me?

Minuchin: You, in relation to him, because it is the way in which you are compensating for what you assume is his authoritarian, rigid parenting. It is the same as if you were saying that you need to be soft because he is too hard.

Mother: Yeah, right.

Minuchin: So something between you two needs to change. (*To husband.*) Can you change her?

Father: I don't know.

Minuchin: That's your job. You need to change her.

Mother: I never really realized that she could think I would back her up against you. You never said that.

Father: She knows that she can come to you for protection.

Mother: I never really thought of her as thinking I would back her up.

With the change in the pattern of transaction among the spouses, there is a change in the perspective of the parents vis-à-vis the daughter. One of the results of a successful unbalancing and change of perspective in a subsystem is its ripple effects throughout the family system. In the measure to which the husband and wife begin to challenge their pattern of transaction and accept the possibility that the wife can develop more effective alternative ways of relating to the husband and that the husband can develop more flexible and nurturant patterns in his transactions with the wife, Patti's position in the implicit interspouse conflict becomes unnecessary. She recedes to being a misbehaving four-year-old, instead of being a field in which the spouses transact their conflicts. As a result, there is a detriangulation of the girl and the appearance of a more effective executive subsystem. In this session, this intervention sparks changes in the pattern of behavior of the mother-daughter subsystem. Therapy continues for two more sessions. Annual follow-ups for three years indicate that the changes in the family have stabilized.

ALTERNATING AFFILIATION

In certain families an alternating affiliation with conflicting subsystems can result in a change in the hierarchical pattern of the family. Affiliating in alternation with both sides is a difficult technique to execute effectively, because the intervention can be framed by members in such a way that it serves to maintain the existing symmetry and distance instead of producing alternatives. Besides, family subsystems in conflict have a quality of inducting the therapist into the "Libra" position of judging and dispensing favors equally, so that the goal of justice is substituted for the goal of unbalancing.

The goal of this technique is to allocate in each subsystem a different and complementary expertise, so that instead of competing for hierarchy in the same context, family members explore new ways of relating in a larger frame. Strategies of this sort are useful in working with families of adolescents, where the therapist supports the right of the parents to make parental decisions and the privilege of the adolescents to question and to request changes in the family decision-making process.

In the Winston family, the 15-year-old son and his parents are locked in a conflict. The youngster thinks that the parents are extremely unfair because they insist that he go to school, come in at a certain hour, and speak respectfully to his parents. In addition, the young man is furious because his parents insist that he keep his room neat, that he make his bed every day, and that he change his sheets once a week. The therapist intervenes by supporting the young man around the issue of his room being his castle. This is the one area of the house over which he should have autonomous control. At the same time, the therapist supports the parents in their desire to have the boy go to school, be respectful to them, and obey ground rules that are for the preservation of his well-being, such as coming in at a reasonable hour.

IGNORING OF FAMILY MEMBERS

This unbalancing technique goes against the grain of the therapist's cultural imprinting, because it requires the capacity to speak and act as if certain people are invisible. The family members who are passed over feel challenged in their most basic right, the right to be recognized. They will rebel against such a basic disrespect by some form of demand or attack. Their rebellion against the therapist can take the form of a direct challenge, but more often it involves a request for other family members to draw closer. This last transaction, which frequently entails a request for a coalition against the therapist, makes a realignment of family hierarchies possible.

The therapist uses this technique in its blandest form when she ignores an overdemanding and centralizing child. When effective, this intervention produces an immediate defocusing on the child, which can have a quieting effect on him. A more active form of this technique occurs when the therapist states her challenge explicitly. She may say, "I don't like to talk with people who don't act their age," or "I avoid children who act like a four-year-old when they are 14; when your daughter becomes 14 again, I will talk to her," or "Isn't it extraordinary how your husband thinks that if he makes a lot of meaningless noise, other people will think he makes sense?"

This type of intervention, in which the therapist talks with family members about the "target" member, can be very alarming because it entails a realignment of family members with the therapist, excluding the targeted member. It can be used with resisting children who challenge the therapy by refusing to talk. The therapist must be able to produce stress in the child by maintaining this inattention throughout the session while at the same time introducing topics that challenge the child.

Patty Dell, a 10-year-old girl, is in treatment because she will not cooperate with her surgeons, who want to perform an operation. For over a year she has refused to talk to her pediatrician. Communication is exclusively through her mother. Patty and her mother have an extremely close attachment. At the initial session, the pull of the family is in the direction of supporting the interdependence between mother and daughter. Patty refuses to talk; her silence makes her mother's intervention mandatory; the mother's style of talking then makes it unnecessary for Patty to talk. The longer the therapist speaks with the mother about Patty, the more he solidifies the status quo. Thirty minutes into the session, Patty is still refusing to talk directly to the therapist.

The therapist then asks Patty's mother to help Patty talk with him: "I want you to try to make Patty talk in such a way that she will talk to me." This intervention represents an important unbalancing maneuver. Since Patty has been silent, it can be assumed that the mother is involved in patterns which keep Patty from talking. On the simplest level, the mother's plethora of words makes it unnecessary for Patty to talk. By asking the mother to get Patty to talk, the therapist changes the nature of the mother-daughter relationship. The child's silence no longer elevates the mother to a position of importance; on the contrary, Patty's reticence now represents the mother's defeat.

The mother accordingly withdraws her support. She distances herself from Patty. The therapist further unbalances the family by telling the mother that she is treating Patty like an infant, not like a 10-year-old. As the mother becomes increasingly stressed, Patty begins to talk for the first time. The therapist continues to unbalance, ignoring Patty and talking to the mother. Patty speaks again, this time louder. But the therapist does not stop talking to the mother.

Minuchin: I'm not talking with Patty because I never talk to people who act younger than their age. Mrs. Dell, I want you to know that I don't talk to people like her. She acts like that because you treat her like a five-year-old.
Patty (loudly): No she doesn't.
Minuchin (to mother): Well, I think you do, Mrs. Dell.
Patty (demandingly): How do you know she does?

Patty is now activated to defend her mother. The therapist therefore speaks with her but maintains the same posture: that the mother is responsible for Patty's acting so young. This gives Patty the opportunity to prove the therapist wrong and defend her mother. She does so by speaking for herself.

The therapist's unbalancing of the system by attacking the mother and making the mother responsible for Patty's behavior distances the mother and daughter. Both his attack and his refusal to allow Patty to talk when she makes her initial forays result in Patty's becoming an active participant in the session, which allows the therapist to separate the two of them more effectively. When Patti is silent, there is only one voice between them—Mrs. Dell's. Any attempt to create a dialog, not to mention distance, between the two cannot be successful.

A more difficult utilization of this technique occurs when the therapist's goal is to change the position of a powerful family switchboard. In a soft approach, the therapist may alternate between the other family members and the switchboard. The therapist ignores and, in a sense, replaces the switchboard by increasing his dyadic contact with the other members and blocking the intrusion of the switchboard. As this technique may endanger the therapeutic system, it must be accompanied by some form of support to the member challenged.

In some families, ignoring a dominant family member becomes a direct challenge. The Koller family, composed of parents in their fifties and an only son, Gil, 17 years old, came to therapy because the son developed anxiety attacks, psychosomatic symptoms, and phobias during his senior year in high school. He also has temper tantrums in which he destroys furniture at home and threatens his parents. In summary, he is an obnoxious young man. The family was in therapy for four months with a competent and forceful therapist who challenged the family pattern of overinvolvement between the mother and son and the peripherality of father. But the therapist felt depowered and helpless as a result of the mother's control of the session and the family pattern that allows the mother to become the third member of any dyad in therapy. The therapist therefore asks a consultant to help break the mother's hold on therapy.

The consultant enters the room after observing the session for fifteen minutes through the one-way mirror. His intervention is a goal-directed one, designed to unbalance the system by excluding the mother in such a way that her centrality in the system will be reduced.

Minuchin (to son): If you go to college, you will depress your mother. Will you do something like that?

Gil: I don't quite understand the point you are trying to make for me. Will you rephrase it?

Minuchin: I think your mother will be very depressed.

Gil: Why will she be depressed? Because she doesn't have me to talk to, or because—

Minuchin: Because she will not have anything to talk about with your father, anything to think about.

Mother: That is not true.

Gil: Mother, let the gentleman speak, please.

Minuchin: I can control your mother. Okay? And I don't need your help. You are a very helpful family, and I notice that you are a very helpful person. What concerns me is that when you realize that you will make her depressed, you will not go to college.

Mother: Well, don't you think I should be consulted, doctor—

Gil: No, that's not true—

Mother: You're talking about me—

Gil: That's not true. It wouldn't bother me that much.

Minuchin: It will not bother you?

Gil: No. You may think that from this short observation, but no, it really won't.

Minuchin: I think so, because, you know, she talks only about you. She watches you—

Mother: Well, that's why we're here, doctor—

Minuchin: She watches you so much. Everything that you say becomes very important—

Mother: Certainly—

Minuchin: And so, what will happen to her?

Gil: What happens to her is her business. What happens to me is my business, and that's my feeling on it.

Minuchin: I don't think you will do it. I think that you will just be so concerned with her that you will—

Gil: No, I won't be. No, I don't mind you saying—I can take what you're saying. You can say whatever you want, but I know that I won't be. That's all I can say. I'm not quite as concerned as you think.

The consultant feels the tremendous power that the mother exerts in the system, her dogged determination that therapy shall be done without changing the usual family pattern. His challenge produces an interesting response from the son, who offers to join him against the mother: "Let the gentleman speak, please." Although the content of this maneuver draws a boundary that excludes the mother, the form of the transaction actually brings her in. The consultant avoids this pitfall by making the exclusion of the mother an operation controlled only by himself. In a family that operates only in triads, he insists on the dyadic transaction. The demand by the mother to be talked to instead of being talked about in her presence is so fair, and so much in accordance with the consultant's ideas about interpersonal respect, that he has to protect himself with an armor of stubbornness equal to the mother's.

Minuchin: Well, I hope you're right, because, you see, your mother doesn't find your father as much an object of interest as she finds you—

Mother: Oh, I—wait a minute. My husband can take care of himself—

Father: Let him say whatever he wants—

Mother: My son is still mine—

Father: Now, easy—

Mother: Well, I'm sorry dear. He's talking about me. I have a right to speak in my own defense.

Gil: No, as a matter of fact, personally that wouldn't bother me, going away to college. You may get that impression from seeing me, but it really won't bother me.

Minuchin: That's my impression, and I think that my impressions are usually correct.

Mother: You are not very modest, doctor.

Minuchin: No, I am not.

Gil: Mom, the point of our discussion isn't the doctor's modesty or not. Let's get back, okay?

Minuchin: Do you think you can train yourself in six months to leave your mother alone?

Ten minutes later, the theme has not changed, and neither has the strategy. Again the mother attempts to recapture her centrality in the therapeutic system, and the husband enters to "recognize" her. Although an episode occurs in which the consultant too answers and "recognizes" the mother, because he cannot avoid responding to a personal challenge, this transaction is short-lived, and the dyad of consultant and son talking about college quickly resumes. The consultant continues the transaction with the son for another five minutes and then begins to talk with the father. This movement is difficult, because not only the mother but now the son as well intrude into the dyad of consultant and father. But the consultant maintains the same strategy of ignoring the mother.

Minuchin: In six months he is going away. Do you think he will be able to be away?

Father: Well, my wife and I have discussed the situation, and we feel that right at the present time he is going through a struggle with himself to overcome the fear of going away.

Minuchin: So, you agree with me that—

Father: Yes, in that respect, I agree with you about going away.

Minuchin: Do you think your wife will let him?

Father: I think my wife will let him go—

Mother: I have not been an overprotective mother.

Minuchin: I think your wife will feel very, very lonely—

Mother: I have John, for God's sake. Why will I feel very, very lonely? I'm concerned about Gil because he is a minor—

Minuchin: When your son is not around, will be you be able to—

Father: I can assure you that we will be able to go on.

Minuchin: I know that you will, because you have your job, and you have your wife.

Father: And I have my son.

Minuchin: Yes, but when he goes out, I think your wife will be depressed—

Mother: That is not so. What makes you arrive at this conclusion, doctor? I mean, what is the basis, I would like to know? You have mentioned this about four times. I would like to know what is your basis for saying that. If you had a basis, I think I am entitled—

Minuchin (to father): That is why I am looking at you, because you have two people here that have difficulties—

Mother: You are presuming that I will have difficulties, Doctor. I mean, that is a presumption on your part.

Minuchin: So, you think that she will be able to make it?

Father: I am sure she will be able to make it—

Mother: I am a self-contained person.

Father: And I am sure that my son will be able to make it, too—

Gil: I enjoy my own company.

Father: I am sure he will be able to make it, providing that he uses his six or seven months that he has to prepare himself, not to play hooky from school, which is something he never did before, and to make an effort just to pass, you know.

Minuchin: It is a very interesting thing. Neither your wife nor your son agrees with me—

Mother: You haven't spoken directly to me yet since you entered the room.

Minuchin: Neither your wife nor your son agrees with me, but I see the immediate future resting heavily on your ability to help these people. I see the possibility of your son not going to college, and it really rests on how you can help both of them. I see you as the key in this possibility.

When the consultant leaves the room after thirty-five minutes, the mother is clearly upset but more willing to accept her husband's and the therapist's views of alternatives. She also is determined to demonstrate that the consultant is wrong. To do so, she becomes less central, less involved with her son.

COALITION AGAINST FAMILY MEMBERS

In this unbalancing technique, the therapist participates as a member of a coalition against one or more family members. This kind of direct participation by the therapist requires, on her part, the ability to confront and to utilize her position of power as the expert in the system to challenge and disqualify the expertise of a family member.

One consequence of this technique is that, although the target member is obviously stressed by the challenge, the family member who is in the coalition with the therapist is equally stressed. His participation in the coalition is predicated on his ability to go beyond the threshold of accustomed transactions and to support the therapist in an open challenge of a powerful member of the family. Since the therapist stays behind after the session, her "ally" in the family needs to be sure that when the family leaves the session, he will be able to "survive" in the new field without the therapist's help. The success of this strategy requires that family members accept the value of the transformation for the benefit of the total family.

Therapists who see the exploitation and damage that parents in dysfunctional families do to scapegoated children may be tempted to rescue the children by creating a coalition with the children against the parents. This type of intervention is usually detrimental for the children, who find themselves without the therapist's support when they are at home. Coalition techniques require a sure knowledge of their stresses for the allied family member.

In another kind of coalition the therapist allies with a dominant family member or subsystem in order to push the subsystem to be effective in its allocated, or natural, function. An example of this intervention is a coalition with parents who are ineffective in establishing executive control over young children. Usually in these families the parents disqualify each other's expertise for controlling the children. A coalition by the therapist with the parental subsystem and against the children binds the parents together and, in effect, detriangulates the children.

The Foreman family, composed of a seven-year-old, grossly obese boy, his divorced mother, and her parents, came to therapy. The structure of the family includes a dominant subsystem of grandfather and daughter, who are overinvolved with each other and with the seven-year-old boy, and a peripheral grandmother. At one session, the family is talking about the way in which they overfeed the youngster. The grandfather and mother, who cannot deny him anything, express their love by giving him food. The grandmother thinks that this approach is destructive for the child.

Minuchin: I would like to sit by the grandmother, because, you know, you are a very wise person. You are really correct, but it is a pity that you are so helpless, because I think that these two people are not letting this young man be even seven. I think perhaps he is three or two. He's big, but he is very, very little, and they are the ones who are keeping him little. It's a pity that, as you are so correct, they don't listen to you. How does that happen, because you could be of great importance to the child? He could grow up to be seven, if you could convince them that you are right.

Grandmother: That's two against one.

Minuchin: But you are right and they are wrong. Even if they are two, you are still right.

Grandmother: Well, I just don't believe in giving a child everything. I don't know, I really don't know, but I tell them about it all the time, and they just say I'm fussing, I'm fussing.

Minuchin: He's seven, but he is really in some ways much younger, and this is because they don't hear you. Can you change seats with your daughter so that you can be near your husband? I think that the one who doesn't hear you is your husband. I think that he is the biggest conflict. If you could convince him, I have the feeling that you could convince your daughter. I have the feeling that you cannot convince your husband.

Grandmother: That's true.

Minuchin: But you know you are right, and I think that they are doing a lot of damage to a child that everyone loves.

Grandmother (to husband): You were damaging the child the other day. It was right at dinner time, remember? I told you we were going to eat dinner very shortly, and you went right on and gave food to him. So many times I told you, "Don't give him this. He don't need that." But no, you are going out and getting him steaks, hoagies, whatever.

The therapist's unbalancing re-establishes the subsystem of husband and wife that had been distanced by the return of the daughter and grandchild and reorganizes the subsystem of mother and child without the grandfather, who has a dysfunctional effect on the mother's executive functioning with her son.

The therapist usually uses a number of unbalancing techniques in succession, ready to change her techniques according to therapeutic need. It is essential in using unbalancing techniques to be sensitive to the system's feedback, which indicates the type of family realignment that has occurred. There are many possible responses by the family to an unbalancing technique. The family members may join against the therapist but nonetheless continue in therapy; the family may terminate treatment; the targeted person may refuse to come to a session; or there may be a family transformation that releases new alternatives to resolve conflicts.

The therapist may have to continue her unbalancing techniques for a number of sessions, maintaining the family in a state of stress. She has to be able to support the family members while she is stressing the system. To do so, she must bring to the system an atmosphere of trust and develop a spirit of collaboration with those family members who are being stressed.

In a session with the Kellerman family, the therapist affiliates with the husband, enters a coalition with him against the wife, blocks the daughter's support of the wife, and finally points out the complementarity of the spouses in maintaining a dysfunctional distance. This family is composed of the parents in their sixties, a 19-year-old daughter, Doris, and a 17-year-old son, Dan, who is the identified patient. The mother complains that Dan is failing in school, disobeys, comes home late, and in general makes it impossible for her to enforce control. Nonetheless, at the first session, when the therapist asks what the problem is that has brought them to treatment, the father takes the position of the patient and defines the problem as his lack of emotional response.

Father: To answer your question why we're here—well, our relationship isn't good, and as a result, or maybe independently, we're having some problems with the children.

Minuchin: Such as?

Father: Such as—well, to speak for myself, I'm not very emotional or don't show much emotion, and very often that is mistaken by other members of the family as not being interested, and that has become a problem. And I don't demonstrate how I feel.

Minuchin: How do you see the kids' response to the problems at home?

Father: Well, the reaction of Doris is to get away from the family; she found outside interests. Dan, he sort of retreated to his own things that would take him smaller distances away—he's interested in biking sometimes; lately it's skateboarding. I think Dan is reacting to his mother. They argue together quite a bit as to what his chores might be or how to do things or when he's to be home. That sort of thing.

Minuchin (to mother): How do you see it?

Mother: He's using his father as a model; he's doing exactly what his father does. You don't know how he feels—no feelings—which to me is a terrible, terrible thing to do to a kid. I think it's terrible. Milt says he doesn't show his feelings, but I don't know whether he has any. I don't know, for many, many years. I had a fantasy one night of him being like a statue, and inside this concrete molded statue was space where feelings were supposed to be, and it was all empty. And outside, you have a concrete statue. Now, I'm very vulnerable to the negative aspects of the relationship, and I'm the one who is having the most reactions, I think.

The definition of the problem presented by both parents seem to be congruent. The father takes over the position of being the problem in the family, even though the son is the identified patient, and the mother describes the behavior of the son as modeled after the father's behavior, thereby making the point that the real patient is the father. Within minutes of the beginning of the session, the therapist is faced with this powerful attack by the wife on her husband, which brings the therapist himself to a critical juncture. Whereas at the beginning of the session, his joining maneuvers made him feel comfortable in the midst of the family, at this point the mother is making a statement that clearly requires on the part of the therapist a response that may unwittingly put him in the camp of the mother. Any tracking on his part of the mother's statement may be construed as an acceptance of the organization of the family wherein the father is peripheral and dysfunctional. Although the father's slow way of talking and the immobility of his face suggest to the therapist that the spouses' assessment of the husband as the patient is correct, accepting this position will support the family homeostasis, keeping the father as the identified patient and the mother as the martyred, helpless, but wanting-to-help wife. It will keep the son as the symptom carrier by proxy and the daughter as the helper in the family. The therapist has to make a decision early in therapy. It might have been useful to hedge until he knew more about the direction of change, but he decides instead to unbalance the family. He governs his unbalancing by the principle of supporting the underdog. He also follows another ad hoc rule in therapy: introduce a cognitive shock by challenging the family member's accepted definition of self.

Minuchin: What you say doesn't make sense to me.

Mother: Why do you say that?

Minuchin: It's literary, metaphoric, but it doesn't make sense. What you are saying is that your style of seeing the world is different from your husband's style of seeing the world and that (*to husband*) she doesn't like your style. The rest doesn't make sense. It doesn't make sense that you don't have feelings. What it is, is that you are different, and you have your angers, your resentments, your pleasures in a style that is different from (*to wife*) yours, and you don't like it.

Mother: But I'm not aware of it—

Minuchin (to husband): She's insisting that you should be like her.

Father: Well, most people are that way.

Minuchin: Yes, but why should you be like her?

Father: I don't try to be like her.

Mother: What about Doris? She said the same thing.

Minuchin: What your daughter said doesn't make sense either. What you are saying is that you would like your husband to be more like you, and that even has music. Rex Harrison in *My Fair Lady* says, "Why can't women be more like men?" (*To husband.*) What she is saying is, "Why doesn't Milt be more like me?" Okay, so you can even put it to music. What is the music in *My Fair Lady*?

Father: It's not a very meaningful song. It's rather a talk song.

Minuchin: Yeah, it's a talk song. Okay, can you remember the tune?

Father: Not the tune.

Minuchin (to wife): Remember that there are many people who are not like you. Different models, different styles.

Father: We are two extremes.

Minuchin: Different, just different.

The therapist enters into a coalition with the husband against the wife. He pays attention to the husband, giving him more space, and he treats the wife lightly and disparagingly. He reframes the wife's complaint as an aesthetic issue and shifts the responsibility for change from the husband to the wife. The danger of this early type of intervention is

that the husband might not accept the coalition, and indeed his first response to the therapist is to insist on his position as a patient ("most
people are that way"). But in his dialog with the therapist, his face becomes more animated, his monotonous way of talking gains inflection,
and it becomes clear that, though depressed, he has a wider possible
range of affect. The therapist contrasts the mother's dream metaphor
with a light metaphor of his own, taking the words of a song and, in effect, setting the wife's dramatic presentation to the music of *My Fair
Lady*. The result of this intervention is to create a structural shift.

Mother: No. Well, it sounds to me like what you are saying is that there
   is a very simple solution to the whole thing. All I have to do is accept
   my husband as he is and that will solve all the family problems. It
   sounds like that to me; it sounds like that's what you are saying to me.
Doris: I don't see the problem as my father being insensitive or unfeeling. Every day I come down I see my brother and mother arguing, and
   then later in the evening they'll argue, and later in the night they'll
   argue over little, little things.
Minuchin (to son): Are these arguments because your mom wants you
   to be different than you are and more like her?
Dan: She's always telling me, "You're just like your father." Most of the
   arguments aren't about that; they're about other things.
Minuchin (to father): Well, I'm wondering, do you see it this way too?
Father: Well, he is more verbal than I am. In my relationship with Bea, I
   don't like to argue and I walk away from it. I'll do anything to avoid
   the argument. But Dan will argue.
Mother: Yes, and I really feel like you said to me, "Look, lady, the problem is you." I just want Milt to be like me, and that's the problem.
Doris: That's one thing everybody wants: people to be like them. Everybody thinks there's something good in them and they can give to everyone else. He's not saying like that's your label and that's what's
   wrong with you and everything else is bad because of that one label.
   You know, you're big, and only one part of you is like that.
Mother: Okay, all right. It's really a big responsibility then, and I'm
   really not up to facing it.

The therapist's intervention produces a change in the family members' position vis-à-vis each other. The mother responds by questioning
first the therapist, then her own position. The daughter focuses on the

mother-brother relationship as a way of moving the problem away from the parents and into the safe arena of the mother-son dyad. In the process, the daughter continues her supportive position to the mother. The identified patient, feeling that the support of the father by the therapist accrues also in his favor, challenges the mother in an affiliation with the father. The daughter then takes a position as translator of the therapist's attack, trying to remove the blaming aspect of the therapist's challenge and support the mother. Although the therapist agrees with the content of the daughter's intervention, to focus or comment on it would detract from the goal of unbalancing. Therefore, the therapist continues with his unbalancing technique, suggesting to the father that he should help his wife.

Minuchin (to husband): Well, I think then that maybe we can find some help. I am wondering how you can help Bea sometimes when she wants things to go the way she thinks they should go.
Father: Well, in the end, it's usually done the way she wants it to go with some or little resistance on my part. Less resistance might help her, or more likely more openness on my part rather than just saying okay, or being more truthful about how I felt about things. I think she enjoys the argument or discussion rather than—
Minuchin: Maybe you better check that out with her and see how she feels.
Mother: I don't know, I don't know what's going on. I know this, I'll tell you this, one of the reasons we're here is because I cannot tolerate living in this situation much longer. I need help then if it's me; then I'm the one who needs help, and somebody is going to have to tell me this and where to go to get it.

When the therapist requests from the husband a helpful position in relation to his wife, he in effect suggests an alternative way of behaving in this subsystem, one that can include the possibility of the husband's helping the wife and of the wife's requesting and accepting the husband's support. This possibility is contrary to the way in which the subsystem has been operating. The husband's first response to the therapist's suggestion is to resume the patient position, but then he considers the alternative way of behaving and adopts the position of the helper. The wife responds to the change, surprisingly, by requesting help from her husband. While this is going on, the daughter brings her chair closer to the mother's chair and puts her hand in the mother's hand in a protective fashion. The therapist challenges the daughter's affiliation without attacking her personally.

Minuchin: Doris, that's not your function. Your function is not to help your mother because you are giving her the message that she cannot handle things on her own, and that's not true.

Mother: I don't know what to do. I don't know what to do. One of the reasons—

Minuchin: If you take your mother's hand, Doris, then you are leaving this empty space between your parents, because your mother holds your hand instead of holding your father's. She could do that if she wants to because your father's hands are available.

Mother: But she reached out to me—

Minuchin: From the beginning you put yourself near your mother, handicapping your father's capacity to move to her and your mother's moving to your father. They have an empty chair between them. Don't sit in it.

Doris: Well, I moved in, and often my mother would say, "Well, that's supposed to come from your father," but I figure that there's a need and it's my mother and I have to do it, and this is one of the reasons why I felt that I had to come back home, to check the situation.

Father: And this is what often happens. I realize I get immobile when she needs help.

Minuchin (to husband): Could you sit in that chair now?

Father: If no one said anything, I wouldn't. (*Sits in the chair near his wife.*) My feeling is that I don't know if I am just being a crutch or if she should be able to handle it alone.

The change in the position of the spouses elicits an accustomed response. Doris operates at this point to reorganize the previous program of affiliation with the mother against the distant, unfeeling, and dysfunctional husband. The therapist challenges the daughter's affiliation, reinforcing the boundaries around the spouses and asking the supposedly immobile husband to make the first move in support of his wife. The husband's response is one of hesitation, reverting to his previous position as a patient ("I get immobile when she needs help"). The therapist helps the father to enact the supportive position by suggesting that he sit in the chair next to his wife. Although the husband in fact moves over, he still is verbalizing his hesitation to make such a big leap in the transformation of the system. This hesitation is not surprising, for the therapist is requesting exploration in an area that is unfamiliar.

Minuchin (*to wife, who sits with her arms flexed, hands closed in tight fists, while her husband has extended his arm and put one hand, palm up, on the arm of his wife's chair*): Look at the way in which you have your hands. And look at his hands. He sends one to you.

Mother: I'm scared to death. I don't know how to react.

Minuchin (*standing up, taking her fist, and opening it*): What about opening this fist and holding his hand?

Mother: It's strange.

Minuchin: You were saying that he should change and he has changed. Now you can change as well.

Mother: Yeah, but it's so far and it's so clear that—

Minuchin: Milt came to this chair, he sat in this chair, he extended his hand, and what did you do? You made a wall here. So don't talk about *his* not moving. *You* are immobile. He opened his hand. Do something in return. He looked at you. *You* didn't look at him.

Mother: I can't stand it.

Minuchin: Oh, then don't say he is not changing. Look at what *you* are not doing.

The wife responds to the therapist's challenge by expressing anxiety. The therapist experiences this as a bid to return to the previous pattern of family organization. At this point, he finds himself in a therapeutic juncture. He must continue stressing the system in order to produce a transformation, but he must also be aware of feedback indicating whether the family members are able to follow him in the exploration of new alternatives in their transactions. The transformation of the system and the family members' exploration of new forms of relating can occur only in an atmosphere of trust in the therapist. If the family members do not experience that trust, they may close ranks against the therapist or refuse to continue treatment. The therapist presents the family members with a restatement of the husband's immobility as an expression of the transaction between spouses ("Don't talk about his not moving. *You* are immobile"). The immobility of both members has been made to look like the immobility of one member by the therapist's elimination of the other member's actions. His strategy produces an increase in anxiety and confusion on the part of the wife.

Mother: I am afraid. I don't know what to do with this. It's like—it's like sitting in a movie and some stranger would put his arm over the back of my chair, you know, one of those creepy people. They come and they touch you and you don't know whether to run and call the usher or whether to sit still and he'll stop or what to do. It's like I don't know him.

Minuchin: You have said that you want more interaction, you want more from your husband and your son, and yet it gives you a funny feeling when Milt moves in your direction.

Mother: In the last five years I said to myself the only way not to be hurt is to try to be more like him, and I did. I tried to be like that. I tried to say, "I don't care. I don't need anybody." But *I* don't want to be like that anymore! I really want to be like I used to be, and then I found that I couldn't, that I have really changed. It's hard when somebody reaches out to you. The normal thing would be to respond. I find that I'm not quite able to do that. It happened before: he touched me and I don't know what to do.

Minuchin: That is saying again that you want to sit on your shit!

The therapist's pressure produces a response in the wife that can handicap the process of change: she begins to assume the position of the patient. An acceptance of this change could release the wife from the necessity of exploring alternative ways of responding to her husband. The mother's description of her anxiety and fear is bait for a therapist. It has a richness of affective components and a suggestion of the possibility of exploring depth. But if the therapist's goal is to effect a transformation in the husband-wife subsystem, his unit of observation and of intervention must be at least the dyad: the mother's lure is a request for a narrowing of the unit of intervention to exclude the husband, producing in that way a maintenance of the distance between husband and wife. The last statement of the therapist ("That is saying again that you want to sit on your shit") is not a challenge to the dynamics of the wife but rather a reiteration of the demand for a transformation of the spouse subsystem.

Mother: But then he'll stick a knife in my back. (*To husband.*) If I drop my defenses when you feel like it, you'll withdraw and you'll start throwing little needles at me, and I don't know when it's going to happen.

Minuchin: Milt, she is throwing you a lot of nonsense. She is saying, "Love me, but don't do it because I will kick you in the balls." She is saying to you, "Hold me," and pushing you away. Don't listen to her.

Mother: Is that true? Is that what I have been doing all these years?

Father: Well, I felt that before, too.

Mother: Why didn't you tell me that?

Father: I'm not a talker, but you push yourself away. I know in the past I felt you preferred to be unhappy.

Mother: I don't know what to say. I don't know what to do next. I don't want to be unhappy like this.

Father: Well, the problem in the past—why I didn't tell you things—was because you get angry when you're criticized. Any kind of criticism on what you are or what you do gets a very strong reaction from you.

The insistence of the therapist on stressing the system in the direction of changing the family members' perspective vis-à-vis each other produces a transformation of the spouse subsystem. The wife now takes the patient position, not as an isolating technique, but as a request for help. This change in the wife is complemented by the response of the husband.

While the parents are talking, the kids talk with each other and then get up and leave the room, indicating that this is a situation in which they are not supposed to participate. This movement is done silently and with an exchange of glances between the children and the therapist, who accepts their boundary-making exodus. The session ends with a change in the self-definition of the spouses. The transformation of the spouse subsystem facilitates the utilization of parts of the spouses' repertory that were unused in their previous transactions.

In this episode the therapist is doubtless unfair to the wife. But once the therapist makes the decision to support the husband, he develops blinders to the "rightness" of the wife's position in the family. She is treated as if she is cause and the husband is effect, which is clearly an incorrect view of the spouse holon. If the therapist had decided to create a crisis in the spouse holon by supporting the wife's view of the husband's immobility, he would in turn have been stubbornly unfair to the husband. The goal of the technique is not be be fair, but to change the hierarchical relation between members of the holon.

When the therapist enters into a coalition with a family member for the purpose of unbalancing a system, her position in the coalition organizes her behavior, and she may lose therapeutic perspective. The only shield that may protect the therapist is a systemic epistemology. She must work with the theoretical and experiential knowledge that the family is a multibodied single organism.

13 Complementarity

The Kellerman family have functioned for many years with an arrangement that the members feel is the *cuadro* of the family. The father is somewhat isolated and the mother somewhat hyper, but they have evolved a style of living together that works. They have areas of shared interest: they are both involved in political issues, like music, and enjoy each other when they visit friends. The daughter, Doris, has grown up as a responsible person, always being a good student, very sensitive to the "vibes" of other people, and close to her mother, in whom she confides and who confides in her when the father becomes too involved in his business. The mother and daughter find support and enjoyment in each other's company, but the daughter is also sensitive to the father's vibes, and she remembers outings with him when she was younger that she enjoyed as a very special treat. The son Dan, who found this threesome arrangement quite tight, developed an interest in sports and has an extra-familial world of friends with whom he shares these "non-Kellerman" areas of interest.

It all worked out well until the daughter finished high school and, searching for a non-Kellerman world of her own, went to Israel for a year to live in a kibbutz. The family organism, proceeding according to its previous rules, recruited Dan to maintain the appropriate distance between the husband and wife. The boy was reluctant to change his extra-familial world for a higher concentration in the world of the family. At this point, when the three-person family organism demanded a transformation from its previous four-person shape, the remaining family members insisted on more of the same. The result was that the mother-son dyad developed conflicts, the son "accepted" the label of the identified patient, the father increased his isolation and guilt, and the daughter returned home to check and repair the system. They then added a family therapist to get out of their mess.

In this fable each member of the family takes a skewed view of the whole. Each one declares, "I am the center of my universe." The father declares, "The problem is probably me, because I am not very emotional." The mother says, "I am very vulnerable to the negative aspects of the marriage relationship, and I am the one who is having the most reaction." Doris thinks, "My mother has a need that I have to fill, and this is one of the reasons I had to come back home." Dan says, "My mother is always telling me, 'You're just like your father.' " The four members see themselves as cause or as effect: "I am the entity—a whole. I contain myself, the present surrounds me and impinges on me. I respond to this context, or I manipulate it, because I am the focus." But it is clear from only one session that four members-as-parts are necessary to maintain the appropriate distance which ensures a style of life that feels harmonious for the family. The actions and transactions of each one of the family members are not independent entities but part of a necessary movement in the choreography of a ballet. The movement of the whole needs four constrained dancers.

"You have to be a delinquent," the judge tells the whore in Jean Genet's *The Balcony*. "If you are not a delinquent, I cannot be a judge." The same recognition of the importance of mutuality and reciprocity is seen in the *I Ching*: "When the father is a father and the son is a son, when the older brother plays his role of older brother and the younger, his role of younger brother, when the husband is really husband and the wife a wife, then there is order."[1] But as Lewis Thomas observes: "The whole dear notion of one's own Self—marvelous old free-willed, free enterprising, autonomous, independent, isolated island of a Self—is a myth: Yet, we do not have a science strong enough to displace the myth."[2] Clearly, the idea of human beings as units remains at war with the notion of the interdependence of all things.

Yet in this war between concepts of the self as a unit and the self as part of a whole, there is a complementarity of opposites. As Fritjof Capra notes, the Eastern mystics become aware that "the relativity and polar relationship of all opposites are merely two sides of the same reality: since all opposites are interdependent, their conflict can never result in the total victory of one side, but always be the manifestation of the interplay between the two sides." The conflict between the ideas of the individual as self and the individual as part of the whole is the result of an unnecessary dichotomization. Niels Bohr tackled an impossible dichotomy when he introduced the notion of complementarity to physics: "At the atomic level, matter has a dual aspect: it appears as particles and as waves. Which aspects it shows depends on the situation. In some situations the particle aspect is dominant, and in others the particles behave more like waves." But the particle and the wave are "two complementary descriptions of the same reality, each of them being only partly correct and having a limited range of application. Each picture is needed to give a full description of the atomic reality and both are to be applied within the limitations given by the uncertainty principle."[3]

If this analogy is carried to family therapy, the self is seen as both a whole and a part of a whole—"both a particle and a wave." "Which aspects it shows depend on the situation." In individual experience, the focus is on the individual as a whole. But when the complementary aspects of the self become parts of a whole, the other parts of that whole, which also are discrete entities, are seen as affecting the behavior and experience of all parts. Beyond the parts, there appears a new entity: an organism, multibodied and purposeful, whose parts are regulated by the rules of the whole. The individual may not experience this multibodied organism, precisely because he forms a part of it. Still, watching a football crowd, one is reminded of Lewis Thomas' observation that "ants are so much like human beings as to be an embarrassment."[4]

One of the therapeutic goals in family therapy is to help family members experience their belonging to an entity that is larger than the individual self. This operation, like the unbalancing technique, aims at changing the hierarchical relationship among family members, but this time by challenging the whole notion of hierarchy. If the family members can achieve a way of framing their experience so that it spans longer periods of time, they will perceive reality in a new way. The patterns of the whole organism will achieve salience, and the freedom of the parts will be recognized as interdependent.

This concept is foreign to common experience. People generally experience themselves as acting and reacting. They say, "My spouse nags me." "My wife is overdependent." "My child is disobedient." From the castle of the individual self, they see themselves as besieged and as responding to that siege. At a session with the Kingman family, composed of the husband and wife and a young psychotic daughter who is almost mute, the therapist asks the girl how long she has been in the hospital, and both parents answer simultaneously. He asks the parents why they answered when he asked their daughter a question. The mother says that the daughter makes her talk. The father explains that since the girl is always silent, they speak for her. "They make me silent," the girl contributes, with a vague smile.

Each of these people has a blind-man-with-the-elephant version of the same reality. Experientially, each of them is correct, and the reality that each defends is the truth. Yet many other possibilities exist in the larger unit.

People in Western culture are constrained by the same sequential grammar. They too tend to see the girl's silence as moving the parents to answer, or the parents' speed as silencing the girl. At one level, everyone knows that these are two sides of one coin. But they do not know how to see the whole coin, instead of heads or tails. They do not know how to "circle around the object and get a superimposition of multiple single impressions" when they are part of the object they must encircle.[5] This requires a different way of knowing.

To facilitate this different way of knowing, the therapist must challenge the family members' accustomed epistemology in three respects. First, the therapist challenges the problem—the family's certainty that there is one identified patient. Second, the therapist challenges the linear notion that one family member is controlling the system, rather than each member serving as a context of the other. Third, the therapist challenges the family's punctuation of events, introducing an expanded time frame which teaches family members to see their behavior as part of a larger whole.

CHALLENGE TO THE PROBLEM

The therapist's first challenge to the certainty of an identified patient apart from context, may be simple and direct. An agitated, depressed patient, Mr. Smith, started the first family session with Minuchin saying, "I am the problem." "Don't be so sure," the therapist told him. The rest of the family agreed with the patient's formulation: "I am the world, and I am the problem."[6] In effect, they were saying, "You are depressed and upset. You alone need help." The family therapist observed the same data, but saw it in terms of how people act and are activated in a system.

Similarly, when Gregory Abbott starts a family therapy session with his wife by saying, "I am depressed," the therapist's first question is not an acknowledgment ("You are depressed?") but a challenge ("Is Pat depressing you?"). Simple questions like this challenge the way people experience reality. They introduce uncertainty.

Therapy starts with a shared consensus of family members and therapist that something is wrong. The family is in therapy because their way of being has failed them, and they want to search for alternatives. Yet because they are wedded to their accustomed truths, they will resist alternatives even while seeking them. The therapist, who occupies the hierarchical position of the expert, may with a simple statement—such as, "I see other factors in the family that contradict your view that you are the patient"—put a different light on the shared experience of an identified patient. The response of the family and the identified patient himself may be to restate their reality that, "He is the patient."

In some families the symptoms are clearly borne by one person, as in psychosomatic families or families with a psychotic member. In such cases the therapist can use the authority of his expertise, stating that in his experience with families like these, the families are always involved in the maintenance of the problem, and are frequently involved in its origin. He may add, "I know you cannot see it that way yet, but stay with me for a little while, just on faith." He may suggest, "Talk among yourselves about the way the family supports or contributes to Janie's problem, because you know more about each other than I do." Or he may treat the situation like a detective story: "You have the clue. I will listen while you explore it."

Sometimes the therapist will challenge by expanding the problem to more than one person: "You have a problem in the way you relate." A parent who brings an unmanageable child is confronted with the reframing, "You and your daughter are involved in issues of control." An identified patient may be described as the family healer, since the family's concentration on him saves the siblings, or as the detourer of problems between other family members. A therapist may work with paradox, introducing confusion into the family reality by suggesting that the symptom should be maintained, since it serves the health of the family as a whole.

All these presentations block the routine response to the identified patient as if he were a whole autonomous entity. The therapist challenges the family presentation of the identified patient as a possessed person. But since the family came to therapy because their ways of dealing with the identified patient have not worked, the therapist only makes explicit what the family members already know.

CHALLENGE TO LINEAR CONTROL

The therapist challenges the notion that one member can control the family system. Each person is rather the context of the other. In the case of the agitated depressed patient, Mr. Smith, the second question Minuchin asked, after "Don't be so sure," was, "If your problems were caused by somebody outside of you, by somebody in the family, who do you think would cause you to be so depressed?" Again, the therapist was not introducing new data. He was introducing a different way of punctuating reality.

The response to the question, "Who is involved with you in a reciprocal relationship that supports your symptoms?" is usually some variation of "I own my illness." Although a person may blame his family for a thousand and one issues, he does not give them the control of his symptom. "I own my depression" is in essence a statement of the integrity of the self. Moreover, only the individual can report the felt experience. To accept mutuality of ownership of a depression would seem to be a surrender of self. Therefore, the therapist tries to induce the recognition of a mutuality of context rather than of ownership.

In the Ibsen family, consisting of a father, mother, and 26-year-old son with severe obsessional symptomatology, the son spends two to three hours in rituals before he can cut a piece of bread. So every night the mother cuts his bread for the next day. The therapist asks the family who composes the music that they all dance to. After some hesitation, the young man says, "I think I do." The therapist suggests that he should move, sitting not between his parents but in front of them, so that he can see how they dance to his music. Later the therapist asks if the son has noticed that his mother is obsessed with cutting bread for him every night. Perhaps, the therapist suggests, he is dancing to her music. This sequential left-and-right attack on the discreteness of self creates havoc in the family's well-formulated concept of the ownership of the problem. Once they have grown comfortable with the concept that the parents dance to the son's music and the son dances to his mother's, the therapist may then want to confuse them further by pointing out how the dance of the mother and son protects the father from involvement.

There is a generic technique for buttressing the concept of reciprocity: the therapist describes the behavior of one family member and assigns the responsibility for that behavior to another. The therapist may say to an adolescent, "You are acting like a four-year-old," and then turn to the parents and ask, "How do you manage to keep him that young?" Or the therapist may say, "Your wife seems to control all the decisions in this family. How did you engineer all of that work for her?" In this technique the therapist is, in effect, affiliating with the person he seems to attack. The family member whose behavior is described as dysfunctional doesn't resist the description because the responsibility is placed on another.

The same technique can be used in signaling improvement. "Now you are acting your age," the therapist may say to the child, and then shake hands with the parents, saying: "Clearly you did something that allowed John to grow up. Can you describe it? Do you know what you did?" By pushing the family to own the change of one of its members, the therapist encourages the system as a whole to accept the notion of the reciprocity of each of its parts.

The individual therapist tells the patient: "Change yourself. Work with yourself so you will grow. Look inside and change what you find there." The family therapist makes a seemingly paradoxical demand: "Help the other person to change." But since change in a person necessitates change in his context, the real message is, "Help the other to change by changing yourself as you relate to him." The concept of causality loses its rough edges of blame in a conceptualization that posits the indivisibility of context and behavior. Both the assignment of responsibility and the consequent allocation of blame recede into the background of a more complex design.

CHALLENGE TO PUNCTUATION OF EVENTS

The therapist challenges the family's epistemology by introducing the concept of expanded time, framing individual behavior as part of a larger whole. Although this intervention rarely achieves its aim of changing the family's epistemology, family members may catch a glimpse of the fact that each of them is a functional and more or less differentiated part of a whole.

In families, an individual may change his behavior for a while without affecting the organism as a whole. For instance, in a lunch session with the family with an anorectic, the parents may alternate between a demanding position and a protective one. But the result is an equal balance, which keeps the child triangulated and noneating.

In the Kellerman family, the husband starts the session as distant, unemotional, and immobile, while the wife requests proximity. When the husband is impelled by the therapist to offer proximity, the wife responds with a phobia about being touched, keeping the previous distance. Individual behavior changes from moment to moment, but the system remains the same.

Traditional psychoanalysis, challenging the notion of willful behavior, promotes the illusion of an internalized context. The interpersonal school, field theory, gestalt, and relationship theories keep the context outside, limiting one's individual freedom without challenging one's individuality. Family therapy, by introducing the self as a subsystem, opens the vista of the individual as a part of a larger organism.

The techniques of introducing an expanded framework are generally of a cognitive nature. The therapist may point out to family members that their transactions are rule-governed, saying: "You have been doing the same dysfunctional dance for ten years. I will help you look at things differently. Maybe together, we can find other ways of dancing."

Pointing out the isomorphism of transactions serves to indicate that the behavior of the family obeys rules which transcend the individual member. For example, in an enmeshed family a youngster sneezes; the mother hands the father a handkerchief for him; the sister looks in her purse for a handkerchief. The therapist says, "My goodness, look how one sneeze activates everybody. This is a family that makes helpful people."

In another case the father disqualifies one daughter a few minutes after all the siblings have jumped on her. "This is a family that makes scapegoats," the therapist says.

The Abbotts are a couple in their thirties who have been separated for a month, the husband having left his wife and two very young children and moved into an apartment to "find himself." Three minutes into the session, the husband responds to a protective statement by the therapist.

Gregory: You seem very compassionate. I feel your warmth, so I feel more comfortable. What's happening with me right now with regard to my relationship with Pat is, I'm feeling less depressed having gone—being out of the house.

This statement is made from the perspective of "I feel your warmth, so I feel more comfortable. I'm feeling less depressed." The husband positions himself at the center of his reality and contemplates a universe that exists only because he is observing it and reacting to it.

Minuchin: Are you saying that Pat depresses you?

The therapist answers with a statement of relationships. Between these two statements there is an epistemological schism. In Gregory's world there is a clear boundary between himself and the surrounding world: if a tree falls in the woods and he is not there, the tree has not fallen. Gregory's reality is what is mapped by his senses and reconceptualized by him. The therapist's question, "Does Pat depress you?" challenges Gregory's epistemology by saying, in effect, "You are not a whole; you are a part of your context." The therapist's statement, couched in necessarily sequential language, is not yet dealing with a holon, but it expands Gregory's universe to include an interactional context: Pat.

The rest of the session revolves around an attempt on the part of the therapist to erode the certainty with which the couple conceives of the reality of their individual relationship by introducing the notion of complementary transactions between parts of a holon.

Gregory: I don't give her that responsibility, you know; I don't lay that on her. I feel depressed and I felt really depressed for some time in the situation.
Minuchin: Hold it! You said you were depressed at home, you left home, and you are less depressed. You are saying that Pat depresses you.
Gregory: No, I really take responsibility for being depressed. I can't put it on her.
Minuchin: For a moment, follow me. You are depressed, and Pat does not help you with your depression.
Gregory: Right.
Minuchin: Why doesn't Pat help you?
Gregory: I guess I feel that a lot of my needs weren't being met. I felt very frustrated. I felt very deprived.

Gregory "owns" his depression like a badge of honor. Married for ten years, he nevertheless considers himself devoid of a family context; neither wife nor children are responsible for or contribute to his depression. The therapist accommodates to Gregory, accepting his wholeness, but suggests a family context for his depression: Pat is not the cause, but since she is not helping him, the void of her response contributes to his condition. Gregory's world is expanded to include at least his interaction with his wife. Gregory's response is a masterpiece of "I feel" statements, but he accepts the fact that he is responding to an impact from outside.

Minuchin: Can you be more concrete? I don't know in what way Pat isn't helping you.

Gregory: We had planned a vacation in Florida in December, and we had a lot of problems dealing with getting away on vacation or arranging for babysitters.

Minuchin: You wanted to have a vacation with Pat alone, without the children?

Gregory: Yes, with Pat alone. The longest we've gone is for three or four days at a time once or twice, and I wanted to take a longer period of time and go to Florida. Like a week.

Minuchin (to Pat): How did you see that enterprise?

Pat: First of all, I want to interrupt you, because we've gone for longer than three or four days and it was ten days you wanted to go. I'm very picky about those things because it's very painful for me to leave the kids at this age, or maybe it will be later on too, and I felt that I was willing to go because he wanted to go and it had been an issue for such a long time. It was just very hard to leave them.

Pat's reality is a reality of responses. Caught between the necessity of allocating priorities to the needs of her children and those of her husband, she feels exploited by his demands. In this family, the spouse subsystem and the parental subsystem, which doesn't include the father, are in conflict.

Minuchin: So, you're depressed also?

Pat: I'm very depressed now. I've been very depressed since he left.

Minuchin: What does Gregory do to depress you?

Pat: He talks about leaving frequently. And I feel that he doesn't want me for me. That he's talking in a very distant kind of way—"I want to expand and enjoy myself, take care of myself, and do exciting things and have a good time, and if it's not with you, it can be with someone else."

Minuchin: I want to force both of you to think concretely. *(To Pat.)* What does he do to you that makes you feel like you want to kick him?

(*To Gregory.*) What does she do to you that makes you feel like you want to leave? Talk with each other about that.

In the painful void of the separation, both spouses increase their *I* view of the world. The therapist requests that each observe the other as a context for self, and he initiates a transaction between the spouses.

Pat (to Gregory): You talk to me as if you are presenting a history of some other family, but I don't get any sense that you really want me. And you talk about wanting certain things in a very arrogant, cocky sort of way, about you getting filled up and you having an independent life; and I want to hear from you, "I want you, I need you," and I don't hear it. I hear you saying, "Let's have some kind of joint therapy," but it sounds very intellectual, very distant, and you are happier and relieved to be away from the situation. I guess I want you to suffer and want me back, and I don't see it.
Minuchin: He has a much easier time. You are with the kids. He doesn't need to be with the kids. He takes himself out and you get all the problems.

Whereas "Pat's family" functions as a complex system, including individual, parental, and spouse holons, both spouses have agreed to keep "Gregory's family" functioning as a simple system, with only individual holons in interaction.

Pat: Well, that's what I resent. I want him to want me so desperately that he is willing to put up with all the hassles and responsibilities and the things he doesn't like because being together would be the only thing that he wants.

In their world of integer selves, neither spouse sees Gregory's self as being a part of the children's context, with obligations and responsibilities toward them. Also in Pat's conceptualization, love doesn't seem to occur in a context between people. It is a feeling that emanates from the lover to the loved, like the warmth of the sun, without expecting anything back. With this concept of reality, there is nothing that she can do to produce change except wanting things to be different.

Minuchin (to Gregory): What are the kind of things about her that would make you feel like she wants you to feel?

The therapist continues avoiding interventions that are related to individual dynamics, instructing the nusband to think about his wife as a context for his own changing.

Gregory: Her fears, her worries about the children if she's away from them, depress me, and that's something that I would like to change. To feel some freedom, so that when we are both together, we are really together, and if we're with the kids, fine, we're really with them. But I don't feel that I have her really to myself when we're alone. It's like the kids are still there because they are still in our minds.

Minuchin: So, you must be doing something that is not exciting to Pat that she needs to take the kids with her when she is with you. Now, what do you do?

Gregory: You know she—

Minuchin: What you are saying is that in some way or other, she finds that being with you is boring, and she prefers the kids to you. Are you a boring person?

Gregory (laughing): I think that's great. I really never thought of it in those terms. You know, I find it's funny.

The therapist interprets the formation of the overinvolved mother-children subsystem as a "result" of the failure of the spouse subsystem. This shift of perspective has a freeing effect on Gregory. Perhaps he could change the relationship of Pat and the children by changing himself in the spouse holon.

Minuchin: Is he a very boring person?

Pat: I wouldn't use the term "boring." But he's not there, is the feeling that I have. He's not there emotionally.

Minuchin: Then you want to kick him back.

Pat: I guess I chronically want to, so it's hard to sort out how much of it is that.

Minuchin: You chronically want to kick him?

Pat: Yes.

Minuchin (to Gregory): How does she do that?

Gregory: I feel her anger often, being irritable, kind of short, kind of stern, matter of fact, and also sexually not available. Tired, getting more tired and going to bed earlier, just not affectionate, not bubbly, or into really being with me. You know, making contact with me.

Pat: Neither are you.

Gregory: I feel especially in the sexual area I approach you very often, very frequently, and I really feel your lack of interest, and it has gotten better at times, but the majority of the time I'm pursuing you.

Pat: And I don't accept your saying that. I think that I've been variable and you've been variable, but I really don't agree that you have been any more available than I've been, and I've been aware of having sexual feelings toward you at times when you've been totally rejecting me and talking about leaving.

Gregory: And I remember we talked about it, how I started turning off when I kept feeling rejected by you.

Pat: And I feel that I kept turning off when I felt rejected by you.

Minuchin: I want you to continue.

The transactional focus moves the couple toward a kind of symmetrical seesawing in which equilibrium is achieved by alternating one-upmanship. The spouses maintain their focus on the individuality of two units responding sequentially to each other. The therapist experiences the couple's signal that they have reached their usual threshold of nonresolution and are ready to move away to a different issue. He keeps them together, hoping that in their stress they may begin to explore alternatives.

Pat: A few weeks ago it really seemed as if things were starting to crystallize when we started talking about how absurd it was because we were both wanting the same thing, to feel love by the other one, and I really started to feel closer to you and found you more appealing and you were softer and I was liking you better softer and you seemed to be wanting affection also, and then that's when we had one more fight and you were just ready to go and you just left.

Gregory: That was one particular day, and I felt you really being motivated and really warm and I let down also. And one little argument did make me feel angry again because of all the things in the past, especially the Florida thing.

Pat: Gregory, it wasn't one day. It was a few days, and then you went on a vacation alone three weeks ago by yourself and that's why it got so cut off at that point.

The wife starts contact by describing the development of a transactional pattern leading to intimacy. She then reverts to a grievance, to which Gregory accommodates by moving to a symmetrical escalation, and the wife accommodates to the husband, and so on.

Minuchin: I have been keeping a score card, and I would give each one of you three points: you are pretty good, you kicked him three times, and you kicked her three times. Since you both tied your score, continue and try to get out of it.

Gregory: I feel confused. I feel very hot right now and anxious and pressured.

The therapist describes the couple's transactional pattern and insists on change in it. The husband counters with a regression to the self as a unit.

Minuchin: You don't understand what I'm talking about. You know, I'm fascinated by the fact that you don't understand something very simple. I am saying, "Do begin to talk with each other in such a way that the other person doesn't feel like kicking you back."

Gregory: I feel like I'm wanting to be accepted by her right now.

Minuchin: She can't. She can't if the only thing that you tell her after kicking her is that you want her to accept you. You need to do better than that. You need to do it in such a way that she should want to.

Gregory: I'm wanting you to remember my softness, my vulnerability, and my loving for you and my loving for the kids, and I'm feeling confused right now. I'm aware of hurting you and I don't like that feeling, and I'm aware of keeping my distance and I don't want you to know that. I'd like to cover it up.

Pat: I am very afraid of you leaving me.

Whereas the spouses' language is still sprinkled with *I* statements, they have accepted the fact that they are the context for each other and that, as such, they can influence their spouse's behavior by behaving differently to that person. The therapist's insistence on the reciprocity of the spouses' behavior and, indeed, the indivisibility of the spouse holon relieves each of its members of the total responsibility for the holon's reality. Both of them, as parts, are needed for maintaining or changing the holon's choreography. Later on the husband talks about a day that he spent with his two children in his apartment.

Minuchin: How did that work?

Gregory: It was a very good experience because I realized that I had more patience and more tolerance with them when I was doing it myself, and I was in control of the situation and they responded to me and I fed them and changed diapers. You know, it was very easy.

Minuchin: You were with both kids?

Gregory: Right. And I wasn't resentful, and I felt that I could take care of them in my own way without her criticism that I will do it wrong.

Minuchin: When you take care of the kids, your wife is your supervisor?

Gregory: Well, if I'd do it my way, and she would say you can't do that, I'd start backing up.

Minuchin: I'm pleased that you had that experience of spending one day alone with your children.

Gregory: I am, too.

Pat: I was, too. I came home that day and I was really very moved by seeing what was going on, and I had the feeling that it is unreal and crazy that we're separated, because he was very soft with them and very involved and stayed for another two hours and we fed them dinner together and played with them together. He said it was because he didn't have any expectations of me, but he was very easy and soft with me and I really felt good with him. But then he left.

Minuchin: He says that he can be a father when he is a father, but he can't be a father when he is your spouse.

Pat: He said since we're separated he feels more like a father.

The organization of this family is such that the spouse and parental holons are conceived as in conflict, robbing from each other. This leaves as a "solution" for Gregory to be a father only when he is not a husband.

Minuchin: And what happened when you were together?

Pat: He just wasn't there. I think it became a cycle. He just went out of the room if the kids and I were there.

Minuchin: It is a cycle in which you participate.

Pat: But he kept saying no, I don't want to spend more time with the kids, and so if we were home with the kids, I was the one that was expected to be with them.

Minuchin: It's also true that you took the kids and spent a lot of time with them when you felt alienated from him, and you (*to husband*) felt that when she was with the kids, she was not giving you anything, but you supported it because it gave you more time for yourself.

The adult members of this family have managed to defend their individuality against the encroachment of the family system with the catastrophic result of being themselves diminished by the process of belonging. In families that find themselves in this or similar situation, it is useful to give a task to the husband to take care of the children for a period of one or two weeks as a way of experiencing the sense of belonging to the parental holon. It is also useful for the spouses to meet with the therapist without the children during this time to develop a sense of belonging to a holon larger and richer than each one of them.

Ernest Frederick Schumacher points out that if man ever wins the battle with nature, he will be on the losing side.[7] Similarly, family members must understand experientially that if they win the battle with the family, they will lose their belonging. To get this point across, the therapist must be able to expand the family members' focus of attention, teaching them to see not a movement, but the whole dance. They must experience not action, response, and counterresponse, but the whole pattern.

14 Realities

A family has not only a structure but also a set of cognitive schemas that legitimate or validate the family organization. The structure and the belief structure support and justify each other, and each can be a therapeutic point of entry. In fact, a therapeutic intervention will always affect both levels. Any change in the family structure will change the family's worldview, and any change in the worldview will be followed by change in the family structure, including change in the use of the symptom to maintain the family organization.

A family coming to therapy presents only their narrowed perception of reality. They may be defending institutions that have lost their utility, but in their worldview, nothing else is possible. They want the therapist to repair and polish their accustomed functioning, and then hand it back to them, as it were, essentially unchanged. Instead, the therapist, a creator of worlds, will offer the family another reality. She will use only the facts that the family recognize as true, but out of these facts she will build a new arrangement. Testing the strength and limitations of the family constructions, she will build upon their foundation a more complex worldview, one that facilitates and supports restructuring.

THE FAMILY'S WORLDVIEW

In 1952, Minuchin was in Israel interviewing a recent immigrant, an adolescent Moroccan girl, who had vague psychosomatic complaints. In the middle of a question her muscles tensed and her eyes widened in terror. She got up, pointing to something or somebody behind my back, and yelled, "Mustafa!" Her panic was so contagious that I whirled around to see what was behind me. She was pointing to a butterfly.

Thinking she was having hallucinations, I turned back, ready to avenge myself by making a diagnosis and prescribing tranquilizers. But she told me that her father, four years before, had died with his mouth open. When that happens, the soul floats out of the body and is transformed into a butterfly. The girl, her family, her village, and the surrounding villages all knew that that was true. Was it real?

Richard Llewellyn describes the trial of a Massai warrior who had killed a white settler because the settler had killed and eaten the warrior's sister. That sister was a cow who, as a calf, had been nursed by the same cow that supplied milk for the infant warrior. Although the lawyer tried to convince the British court of the reality of kinship between the warrior and the cow, the warrior was found guilty.[1]

Llewellyn's descriptions of the Massai are extremely vivid. My son and I were so impressed with this book that for a while, in moments of recognition and respect for each other, we would spit on the floor and say, "I see a Massai," in what we thought was true Massai fashion. Spitting, a symbol of respect in desert countries, has, of course, a very different meaning in our culture. But is the reality of the British law more real than the reality of the Massai?

Sol Worth and John Adair, who were interested in finding out what people see, as opposed to what they say they see, trained a group of young adult Navajos to use a movie camera.[2] Their film seemed to me to be a disconnected series of shots: a loop, a road, horses, trees. For Navajos, it all connected with a Navajo myth of twins. In the late 1960s, Richard Chalfen and Jay Haley developed a similar project. A group of inner city black adolescent girls wrote a script for a movie, in which all of them acted. The result was a family drama showing arguments, drunkenness, caring, closeness, and a vivid human immediacy. In the same project, a middle-class white group produced a movie with wide lens shots of the sky, scenery, houses, and long shots at objects rather than people. Which view of the world is correct?[3]

What is reality? What is a rose? One could paraphrase Gertrude Stein and declare that a rose is a rose is a rose, hoping that repetition would bring intensity, redundancy, and truth. But does everyone see the same rose?

Ortega y Gasset writes of reality: "This ash tree is green and is on my right . . . when the sun sinks behind these hills, I shall follow one of the ill-defined paths open like an imaginary forest in the tall grass . . . then the ash tree will go on being green, but . . . it will no longer be on my right . . . How unimportant a thing would be if it were only what it is in isolation. How poor, how barren, how blurred! One might say that there is in each thing a certain latent potentiality to be many other things, which is set free and expands when other things come into contact with it. One might say that each thing is fertilized by the other; that they desire each other as male and female; that they love each other and aspire to unite, to collect in communities, in organisms, in structures, in worlds. . . The "meaning" of a thing is the highest form of its coexistence with other things . . . that is to say, the mystic shadow which the rest of the universe casts on it."[4]

Reality thus seems to be the rose, or the ash tree, *plus the order in which you and I arrange them*. It is the meaning we give to the aggregate of facts that we recognize as facts. And there is one more step. Reality has to be shared with others—others who validate it.

DEVELOPING A WORLDVIEW

This socially validated worldview frames the reality that frames the person. The individual, in learning very early in life to apprehend the reality that is presented to her as objective, develops the filtering lenses that will be with her throughout life. Those who convey this reality to the infant, Herbert Mead points out, are "significant others," who impose on him their definition of the situation: "The individual experiences himself as such, not directly, but only indirectly from the particular standpoint of other individual members of the same social group or from the generalized standpoint of the social group as a whole to which he belongs. . . It is the social process itself that is responsible for the appearance of the self; it is not there as a self apart from this type of experience."[5]

Mead no longer focuses on a simple linear cause and effect, but on feedback. He is concerned with the dance. His is an organismic view: the self in context is also part of the context of the self's significant others.

Harry Stack Sullivan applies Mead's concepts of the dialectic exchange between self and context in his theories of interpersonal psychiatry: "The facilitation and deprivation by the parents and significant others is incorporated into the self. . . . Since the approbation of the important person is very valuable, since disapprobation denies satisfaction and gives anxiety, the self becomes extremely important. It permits minute focus on those performances which are the cause of approbation and disapprobation, but very much like a microscope, it interferes with noticing the rest of the world."[6]

Starting with the influence that significant others have on the child, Sullivan recognizes that the early self is a creation of self plus context. But hampered by the restrictions of an individual, linear paradigm, Sullivan moves away from the self in context to postulate the internalization of the significant others. It is as if the dance of life becomes introjected and can no longer encompass the continuing transactions with significant others in the task of reality construction.

How individual reality is constructed can be studied by looking at the way the context becomes internalized; or one can approach from the opposite direction, dealing with the way societal institutions affect the individual. Both points of entry present a problem at the interface. Sociologists remain too distant from the specific reality of the individual, addressing themselves only to the homogenized reality of the institution. Individual theorists get stuck in the tremendous idiosyncratic complexities with which an individual transacts in context. And both approaches may lose the rhythm of the dance.

To explore the organismic characteristics of the individual in context requires a smaller institution. The family is the matrix in which societal rules are tailored to the specific individual experience. The family therapist, therefore, is at the appropriate distance for exploration of the system of individual and societal context, without having to separate too far from either element. Being close to the specificity of the individual family members' experiences, but still having the system vantagepoint of the group, the family therapist can encompass the individual and the family holons as whole and as part.

VALIDATING A WORLDVIEW

The way the family develops its structure is analogous to the process by which society develops its institutions. So, too, is the way the family validates its structure. Thus the way in which society legitimizes its institutions gives the therapist a paradigm for understanding how the family's worldview is maintained, and how it can be challenged in therapy.

Peter Berger and Thomas Luckmann distinguish four levels of legitimation of societal institutions, a schema which is useful for the study of family validation. Level one is simple vocabulary, or the presentation of reality through language. A child learns that the thing she is holding is a spoon. This is rock-bottom reality, "the foundation of self-evident knowledge on which all subsequent theories must rest." Level two of legitimation contains simple explanatory schemas that give facts their meaning. These schemas are "highly pragmatic, directly related to concrete action." Proverbs, maxims, legends, and folk tales are typical of this level. Level three of legitimation contains explicit theory, based on a differentiated body of knowledge, which provides the frame of reference for conduct. Because of its complexity, it is transmitted by specialized personnel. The fourth level of legitimation is the symbolic universe, which integrates different provinces of meaning into a totality.[7]

Each of these levels has an analogy in the development of a family worldview, and each offers a therapeutic point of entry for challenging the family validation of reality. The challenge need not be a confrontation. Instead, it may be a shift, or an expansion, which adds to rather than disqualifies what the family is accustomed to.

At level one, basic vocabulary, the therapist pays close attention to the way the family uses words and to the words that are important to them. But the therapist knows that the meaning of words is related to the family context. In a family where love is highly valued, the therapist says to a family member: "You are a prisoner. Your jail is love, but it is still a jail." At this point the word *love* takes on a whole new meaning for the family.

Level two of legitimation, explanatory schemas, includes in family terms the myths and family history that organize both present and future. In families, the members are seen by each other in set ways, and these views endure, even though the reality as seen by the extrafamilial observer may be quite different. The therapist does not have to challenge the family myths outright, but she may rearrange them or expand them, for example by explaining to a child whose father is billed as all-powerful that true respect for such a father implies and dictates the need to disagree.

Level three of legitimation is the body of knowledge entrusted to experts. The family therapist assumes this expertise and possesses the credentials to frame the normal and the deviant in family terms. A therapist's interventions have the support of a body of theory and a professional group.

Level four of legitimation deals with the universal issues of the family's intersection with the larger world. This includes the universals of life, such as that family members are born, grow, and live in social contexts, and that they are independent and also belong to family holons imbedded in larger holons. These universal realities can be used by the therapist to challenge the loyalty that family members have to their own idiosyncratic reality.

CHALLENGING A WORLDVIEW

Validation inevitably raises the related issue of deviance. Legitimation is in fact an ongoing dialectical process. As Berger and Luckmann remark, most societies do not accept a monolithic validation, so that there is a constant interaction of alternative definitions of reality: "Most modern societies are pluralistic. This means that they have a short core universe taken for granted as such and different partial universes co-existing in a state of mutual accommodation."[8]

The family's short core universe gives the family members the security of inhabiting a known territory. Unfortunately, it may also impose limitations that do not have to be there. It sends family members to the defense of flags that they do not really support, and to the attack of bastions that are not really manned by their enemies. Worse, it keeps them in ignorance of things that they know, or could know, inhibits their curiosity about the world they inhabit, and prevents them from exploring worlds they could populate.

The therapist seeks to present some of the different partial universes that are outside of the family's short core universe and which the family members are closed off from. She knows that the family reality is interpreted by its members from the perspective of the holons they inhabit. Therefore, the interpretation of the transmitted universes, and of deviation, is a matter of perspective. And perspective can be changed.

When my children were young, I used to tell them bedtime stories in which a child, named Yankele Mehesforem, visited different countries with their different rules, customs, and myths, and tried to interpret these cultures through the eyes of an American middle class child. The stories were full of the humor of the clash of cultures and the confusion when one reality challenges the truth of another. For the plot, I drew from my experiences in different countries. What I was trying to do with my stories was to introduce my children to a pluralistic view of reality. This is the view the therapist must also learn, so as to offer the family alternative worldviews.

Alternatives should not be framed as another world; people are afraid of new things. Besides, few would abandon, like an old shoe, a reality that has served well, and which has many legitimations supporting it. Instead, the therapist offers, en passant, an expansion—a hint of an alternative—something that modifies the boundaries of the known. The therapist has a variety of techniques with which to challenge the way a family legitimizes its structure. These techniques are the use of cognitive constructs, the use of paradoxes, and the search for strength in the family.

To sum up, I cannot resist sharing the remarks of Captain Mallet at the annual convention of the Identity Club: "Gentlemen, this is an historic moment. For more years than I can remember we have spent our lives in the seclusion of our London quarters toiling at the great theory which is the unifying factor of our lives. It was ever our belief that this theory could be perfected best in isolation: we have known from experience that once a theory is exposed to the knockabout of daily life it loses the bloom on which its beauty depends. Most clubs—and there are many nowadays—ignore this precaution; they pitch their theory into the outside world against all rivals, thus leaving it dependent upon nothing but the hysterical pugnacity of its supporters. This is all very well, but it has always seemed to us that as all clubs are closed circles, permitting no deviations whatever, it is senseless to expose loyal members to the rough-and-tumble of debate. Why argue with a member from another club when we know that both he and you are so inextricably identified with opposing theories that for either to yield a point is like losing an arm or leg? No, gentlemen, since it is the aim of every club to be the only club and of every theory to be the only theory, the way of *our* club is surely the best. We actually do live in isolation from the world—which is to say that we live in exactly the same way as all other clubs except that we do so more comfortably and don't have to pretend that we have open minds. Our beloved theory, the only true one in the world, is the only one we want to hear about. Identity is the answer to everything. There is nothing that cannot be seen in terms of identity. We are not going to pretend that there is the slightest argument about that... We of this club excell all other clubs in that we give our patients the identities they can use best. We can make all sorts of identities, from Freudian and Teddy Boy to Marxist and Christian.

"And what we like about ourselves is the frank way we go about our work. Other clubs stubbornly deny that they try to supply their patients with new identities. They insist that they merely reveal an identity which has been pushed out of sight. Thank God, gentlemen, we shall never be like them! We are proud to know that we are in the very van of modern development, that we can transform any unknown quantity into a fixed self, and that we need never fall back on the hypocrisy of pretending that we are mere uncoverers."[9]

15 Constructions

The family has constructed its present reality by organizing facts in a way that maintains its institutional arrangements. There are alternative ways of seeing, but the family has chosen a certain preferred explanatory schema. This schema can and should be challenged and modified, making new modalities of family transaction available.

The therapist begins by shaking the rigidity of the preferred schema. He also dismisses many of the facts that the family presents, selecting the "therapeutic reality" in accordance with the therapeutic goal. This is a heavy responsibility; the therapist must recognize that his input organizes the field of intervention and may change the family explanation of their reality. The concept of interpretation detours around this responsibility, framing the therapist's task as merely exploring the truth. But when the therapist's position within the therapeutic system is examined, this more comfortable framing is no longer possible. The family's reality is a therapeutic construction.

The therapist's freedom as a constructor of realities is limited by his own biography, by the finite reality of the family structure, and by the idiosyncratic way the family has developed its structure. The therapist is therefore a constrained changer. The family has the capacity to control him by determining his complementary responses. It may also induct him into supporting the family reality. Nevertheless, his input is a factor in defining this field.

There are a variety of techniques to carry the message that families and family members have more alternatives available to them than their preferred modes of transacting. The goal is always the conversion of the family to a different worldview—one that does not need the symptom— and to a more flexible, pluralistic view of reality— one that allows for diversity within a more complex symbolic universe. The techniques of changing the family reality fall into three main categories. They are the utilization of universal symbols, family truths, and expert advice.

UNIVERSAL SYMBOLS

With this technique, the therapist presents his interventions as if supported by an institution or consensus larger than the family. He therefore seems to deal with objective reality.

With some families it is possible to decree that a moral order—god, society, decency, or whatever—prescribes the right way. Ivan Nagy's exploration of mutual commitment among family members falls into this category of intervention, in which the therapist assumes a moral position and becomes the representative of morality.[1]

In the West family, who came to therapy because the father, a minister was having difficulties controlling his two adolescent daughters, Mr. West refers to his wife and daughters as "the three girls." The therapist rises, "stopping the clock," and points up a moral: "You must have difficulties in your relationship with God, since you don't understand that He created hierarchy in the family. There is a right place for the parents and a right place for the children." By choosing universal constructs that fit with the family worldview, the therapist suggests a rearrangement of holons.

The therapist can do the same thing by drawing on common sense or common experience. "Everybody knows" there is a certain shape to things; reaching agreement on the shape is not necessary. There is a time to be playful, and a time to work. Older children are expected to be more responsible than younger. In some families, it is useful to point out that, "since you are older ... younger ... the oldest daughter ... the breadwinner ... you should ... and the rest of the family should ..." The therapist brings the power of group persuasion to buttress his ideas.

It is also useful to decree that tradition prescribes a certain course. Every society trains its people to respond to the magic of correct sequences, and every individual has experienced order in his own development. Therefore, constructions that are built on temporal rituals may partake of the power of magic in effecting transformation.

The power of universal constructions resides precisely in the fact that

they deal with things "everybody knows." They do not bring new information; they are immediately recognized as common reality. The therapist uses this consensus as a platform on which to build a different reality for the family.

In the Mann family, the family reality is that a 28-year-old son Bill,
who has been working abroad for the last five years, returns home with a
psychotic episode of agitated depression, apparently triggered by a
friend who conned him out of $1000 in a relatively simple deception in-
volving oil and Arab shieks. The rest of the family—his parents, Paul
and Mary, and his 23-year-old brother, Rob—respond with concern,
protection, and anxiety to the disorganized behavior of the identified patient.

The dysfunctional structure is the overinvolvement of the family
members, especially the father-older son holon. The son relates to the
father with a loyalty and respect bordering on awe, but also with a deep-
seated and unexpressed resentment. The mother and younger son cannot modify or indeed participate in the overinvolved dyad.

The therapeutic construction, arrived at in the initial session, focuses
on the acute symptomatology of the identified patient. The therapist
normalizes the identified patient by explaining and justifying his behavior in terms of the universal meaning of growing up: a narrowing of alternatives and a partial dying. The therapist then suggests a mourning
ritual to shed the old self and accept the new reality as an older person.
The younger brother and the mother are given specific functions in the
ritual, while the father is kept apart. The construction supports a modification in the family structure, strengthening the differentiation of the
older son, the development of a sibling holon, and the distancing of the
overinvolved father.

Minuchin (to Bill): How are things? Your father called me yesterday
  about you. Today, your mother also talked to me on the phone because they are concerned.
Bill: Well— (*Starts to cry.*) I don't want to be upset. (*Looks at father,
  who is also crying.*) I'm sorry, Dad, really. I'm sorry. I don't wanta—I
  don't know how to get it out. I'm sorry— (*Continues to sob.*)
Father (crying): That's all right. No problem.
Minuchin (to father): Paul, if you cannot be helpful, then you go out of
  the room. It is not right for Bill to be concerned with you if he wants to
  cry, because then he cannot be free. Bill has some need, or some wish,
  to cry at this point, and he should be free to cry without being con-

cerned with protecting you. (*To Bill.*) So go ahead, cry. If you need to cry, cry—and when you have finished crying, we can talk. But go ahead and cry. (*To wife*). Why must Paul cry?

Mother: Well, he's that way.

Minuchin: That's very unhelpful, as you can see, because then your son finds himself involved in protecting Father. There are times in which people feel like crying. Do you feel like crying sometimes, Rob?

Rob: Sometimes I do. Not too often, though.

Minuchin: Well, you are a young chap. How old are you?

Rob: Twenty-three.

Minuchin: What are you doing now?

Rob: Going to school at the university.

The therapist begins with a construction about the freedom to cry. Crying is framed as a right that people have. He challenges the father's constraining effect on Bill, normalizes crying as a wish or a need, and by giving Bill permission to cry, implies that the crying is under the therapist's control. The therapist then turns away from Bill and talks with Rob about neutral issues, waiting for the crying to diminish so he can return to Bill, which he does a few minutes later.

Minuchin: Bill, how long have you been back home?

Bill: Three weeks.

Minuchin: And you have been a year in Venezuela?

Bill: I've been in Venezuela all told maybe two years off and on.

Minuchin: Where in South America besides Venezuela?

Bill: In all of South America, I was working in Colombia, Equador.

Minuchin: Do you speak Spanish?

Bill: Yeah.

The conversation continues in Spanish for five minutes, during which Bill says that he was burned in a business transaction with a "friend." Although he knew that he was being taken, he invested $1000 because he did not know how to get out of the situation. The therapist uses the opportunity to speak Spanish as a boundary-making maneuver, increasing his proximity with the patient and separating the patient from the family. Then Bill begins to cry again.

Minuchin: I want Bill to cry when he needs to cry, and then when he is feeling able to talk, he talks again with me. Paul, what do you think is going on with your son?

Father: His family means everything in the world to him. In my opinion, though—I don't know if my wife agrees—he would do anything for his family. (*Begins to cry.*)

Minuchin: Then why are you crying? I would like you to leave the room, and return when you can organize yourself. (*To wife.*) Your men tend to cry easily, don't they, Mary? (*Father gets up to leave. Bill extends his arms as if to stop him, but therapist blocks the movement. Bill then sits down sobbing.*)

Mother: They are softies, that's why.

Minuchin: Okay. You see, I need to have some people with whom I can talk. Neither Paul nor Bill is able to communicate, so I wish you could move here so I can talk with you, Mary. (*Mother takes the seat husband has vacated.*) Bill, you cry until you are ready to talk with me. Mary, what's your idea about what's going on?

Mother: I think that he was mentally burdened. He got this wonderful job six years ago, and he was always traveling.

The therapist increases the intensity of his construction about freedom by sending the father out and supporting Bill's crying while labeling the father's crying as deviant. The therapist continues talking with the mother and Rob.

Minuchin: Rob, you can invite your father to come back if he can. Tell him that if it will be stressful, I prefer he should not return. (*To Bill.*) Are you ready?

Bill: Yeah.

Minuchin: I feel that sometimes people need to cry. So whenever you feel like crying, you cry, and then I will talk to them and talk with you later.

Bill: Okay.

Minuchin: I still don't understand what your situation is at this point.

Bill: I'll explain—

Minuchin: But when you need to cry, you cry, and I will move to them.

Bill: Okay. About a month ago—no, about six weeks ago, I was in the office and I had a lot of pressures—maybe self-imposed—well, one day I went into the office and then all of a sudden it was like something snapped in my brain. I don't know what it was, but it just snapped (*begins to cry*), and after that day—

Minuchin: If you need to cry, you cry. Okay? I will come back to you whenever you get— (*Turns to talk to mother.*)

Bill: I just—

Minuchin: No, no, no, I don't feel you can.

Bill (taking a deep breath): I'm okay.

Minuchin: Okay.

Bill: And then all of a sudden there was like a sense of unreality. I became disoriented. I couldn't sleep, and like I would take a trip— (*Begins to cry again.*)

Minuchin: Rob, maybe you can get some tissues from the front desk. (*To Bill.*) You just relax, and I will come back to you. I want you to cry until you are finished.

The therapist turns away from Bill and talks with the rest of the family members. He has normalized crying: it is an event that handicaps talking, but it can be accommodated to by waiting. He has also placed the control of crying on Bill while reducing the symptom's effect within the system. Five minutes later, while asking Rob if he has a girl friend, the therapist sees that Bill is listening again.

Minuchin: Bill, do you have a girl friend?

Bill: No.

Minuchin: Did you ever have a girl friend?

Bill: Yeah, I had a couple.

Minuchin: For how long?

Bill: Well—for a few months. You see, my job doesn't provide me the opportunity to have a steady girl friend because I was always traveling.

Minuchin: When you say you were always traveling, what does it mean?

Bill: I would travel every two weeks of every month. For the first year or fifteen months, I was in Latin America. Then I was transferred to the Far East and Australia, and then I would travel—

Minuchin: The Far East and Australia! My goodness, that's quite spread out.

Bill: Then I spent two and a half years in the Far East traveling all the time.

Minuchin: That was also every two weeks?

Bill: Oh, sometimes I would be in a place for a month and a half.

Minuchin: You don't have a home then.

Bill: Here. That's my home.

Minuchin: You don't have any home. You have been five years away from here and you have not established any roots in any other place.

Bill: Yes.

Minuchin: How old are you now?

Bill: Twenty-seven. (*Begins to cry.*)

Minuchin: Okay, I'll come again to you. I want to talk now about something else.

The therapist talks with the family until he observes that Bill has stopped crying.

Father: Doctor, can't you let me say one thing about what happened the last time he was home—

Minuchin: No, no, I don't want you to talk about Bill when Bill cannot talk about himself.

The therapist thinks that although the depressive episode was triggered in Venezuela, the symptomatology is at this point maintained by the close reverberation between son and father. The therapist does not have much information about their dysfunctional transaction, but he operates with a rule of thumb: challenge overinvolved structures. This boundary-making technique is repeated to support the therapist's message that the identified patient has resources that he has not yet utilized fully.

Bill: The only thing is—

Minuchin: Are you ready?

Bill: Yeah.

Minuchin: Are you certain, because if—?

Bill: That's all right. One day I walked into the office and this thing in my mind just snapped and then I had like a sense of unreality, disorientation, and I couldn't sleep, and one night I was coming home from work with a friend and I wouldn't let him leave me, and then my mind spilled out and then I was running around like—

Minuchin: Okay, do you want to stop?

Bill: I couldn't control myself—it was like I was outside my body, you know, and I just—my mind just spilled out like—you know—I didn't know where I was. I have this feeling, this constant feeling of not being able to control myself. I have a sense of unreality. I know I'm at home, but I can't—I have a constant pressure inside my mind—it's like a knot—just this constant pressure. At night I can't—everything begins to choke me like, and I have pains in my—I get constant pressures here, and I just can't sleep and can't—I'm not myself. I just want to feel normal.

Minuchin: No, you cannot become normal yet, because first you need to face some realities about yourself that are connected with this experience. Your sense of trust of yourself has been shattered. Maybe you need to take a second look in the mirror. (*Gestures toward the one-way mirror.*) You have been having a strange idea of who you are, and this guy made you look like a schlemiel, and you don't like that a bit. So, you are feeling now a tremendous sense of uncertainty.

The therapist takes an event in the description and makes it the initial step in a series of constructions that will build on each other to challenge the depressive psychotic organization of the identified patient's reality. This process is carefully planned: the therapist starts his challenge to the identified patient's reality by asking him to look at his image, narrowing his focus of attention to what the therapist will tell him about himself.

Bill: Yes, and I think of crazy things and I can't—I don't know where I am, really, you know, and it frightens me—

Minuchin: Yes, that happens with people at the point in which their sense of trust in themselves is shattered. They go back home and, because you are an adult, you don't find your own place at home either. It is true you are a close family, but this is not your home. For the past five years, you haven't had one.

Bill: I want to make it my home now.

The identified patient's reality of frightening ghosts is not challenged, just explained in terms of accepted "objective" facts known by everybody.

Minuchin: What you are describing is a sense that your old life has been shattered, and now you want to create a new life. But you cannot do that quickly. First you will need to cry for the last five years—for the opportunities you didn't have, for the friends you didn't make, for the dreams that didn't come true, for your being conned probably more than once and not only this time, for the hopes that you thought you would have, for the girls that you didn't go out with, for the friends that you almost made but didn't. I think you need to cry for them and I think you are crying for that. You are crying for your life as if these last five years were a waste, and if that's how you feel, you need to cry. You know, I could give you some pills to calm you, but I am concerned that if I give you these pills, you will not cry. I want you to cry.

The therapist introduces a universal construction. Everyone has "a road not taken." The therapist does not have much information about this patient, but he knows that the sense of missed opportunities is there. He builds his construction carefully from the specific facts that the patient has given him, ensuring that the patient will recognize his own reality. At the same time, the therapist uses a quasi-ritualistic repetition that establishes both proximity and authority, facilitating the patient's acceptance of the suggested task.

Minuchin: I am going away for four days and I want to see you again on Monday. For the next four days, I want you to stay home in your room. Have you ever had a relative that died?
Bill: Yes, my grandfather.
Minuchin: Did you sit Shiva [a Jewish mourning ritual]?
Bill: Yes.

Again the therapist builds into his universal symbolism elements of the patient's life that will make this prescription feel specifically related to the patient's reality.

Minuchin: I want you, for four days between tomorrow and Monday, to sit in your room. You can read, but mostly I want you to cry and to remember your last five years and cry for every opportunity in which you had hopes and you let it drop. Do you understand what I want? I want you to look back at your life and look again in terms of what you could have developed that you didn't. I want, very, very carefully, that you should see that you could have created a home or a friend in Venezuela and you didn't, that you could have had a girl friend that loved you in very special ways in Australia and you didn't, and I want you to think that all of these are missed opportunities, and I want you to go over carefully—four days is not too much to remember five years. Here and there, when you feel that you need to tell something to somebody, I want you to call Rob. Not your father or your mother, because they are too old, but Rob. Rob, do you have classes tomorrow?
Rob: Yes.

Minuchin: And on Friday?

Rob: No.

Minuchin: Can you skip the classes tomorrow?

Bill: I don't want him to miss them.

Minuchin: I am not asking you. This is a prescription. Can you miss the class tomorrow, Rob?

Rob: Yes.

Minuchin: I want you to stay home, also. Don't enter into Bill's room except when he asks you to. Do you have the same room, or what?

Rob: No, I have a room of my own.

Minuchin: So, Bill, you will know that in the house Rob is there, available—because that is important—at any point in which you want to tell about an experience that happened that you had three years ago, two years ago in Australia, in New Zealand, and you will listen, Rob. You will be sympathetic, and he will cry. You will not make any attempt to stop him from crying, because I want him to cry. It is important that you should think about these missed opportunities and feel sad, and it's important that Rob should respect that. He should respect your need to feel sad. You see, I think that in your family they don't respect people's privacy, the privacy of being sad, the privacy of being ashamed because you are so shamed. You are embarrassed, and this is perfectly okay. People should have that right also; people should have the right to feel sad, to feel embarrassed, to feel crazy sometimes.

The therapist organizes the rest of the family around the mourning ritual. The mother is to go out and buy a bottle of good whiskey and, like a traditional Jewish woman in these rituals, prepare food and drink. She is also given the function of keeping the father busy and away from Bill and his pain, since the father's sharing handicaps Bill's crying. And Rob will be available and sharing when needed. This ritual is organized around the reality of one member, since the intensity of his symptom requires an immediate response. Nonetheless, the participation of the family around the identified patient, sharing within the therapeutic system the therapeutic construction, creates a changed family field, separating the father from the identified patient and supporting a sibling holon. In the therapist's experience, these mourning rituals are self-limiting. Patients may spend one or two days crying, then stop. By Monday, Bill, though still quite anxious, is less depressed and more organized.

In the second session, after discussing the way in which the task was implemented and the new proximity that it produced between the siblings, Bill expresses the feeling that, because his parents are so generous, he has to inhibit his wishes or else his parents will immediately fulfill them far beyond his needs.

Bill: I have to sort of restrain myself because if I say to my father—just as an example—"I like that tie," he'll buy me a tie in fifteen different colors. Therefore I won't say, "I like that tie."

Minuchin: Do you really mean that?

Bill: Yeah. And if I like a suit, he'll buy me five suits. So therefore I don't say I want anything. If I ask for a bottle of Scotch, he'll buy me a whole case or four bottles or three bottles. So it loses its meaning. Do you see what I mean by overindulgence?

Minuchin: Of course.

Bill: I think that it doesn't make me feel free to ask them for anything, because whatever I ask them for, they'll overdo it. So then I just do without.

Minuchin: I am very impressed by what you just said. First, because you are very perceptive. The other thing is that I see you as a prisoner. You know, your jail is love, but it is still a jail. It is mutual love, but it's a jail. You cannot have a wish because then you will get it in spades. Then you are a prisoner; you cannot receive.

The therapist, whose goal is to help the identified patient differentiate himself from the family and increase his distance from the father, introduces a metaphor to convey the inhibiting effect of indiscriminate generosity and loyalty.

Minuchin: Let me talk with your father for a moment, okay? Can you allow me, because what you said bothers me a lot, and I just don't understand that. (*To father.*) Is what Bill says true?

Father: To a certain degree. There's nothing in the world I wouldn't do for my children and my wife wouldn't do for our children. We are the way we are, and if the children are victims of the way we are, we'll try to change. The last few days that Bill was in the house, I tried to stay as far away from him as I possibly could. It was very hard. I hope you realize that if you have the kind of love that we think we have, it's very difficult to see your child in this condition. I tried to buy him a suit because he doesn't have any clothes that he wears. He wears the same stinking shirt all the time, and he can go to my closet and have what he wants—

Minuchin: Did you buy him anything?

Mother: We haven't bought him anything since he's been away.

Minuchin: Very good. Okay, good, because the issue is—

Father: The shoes he's wearing are my shoes.

Minuchin: Bill, can I see them?

Bill: Yeah. (*Takes off one shoe and gives it to therapist.*)

As the therapist is dealing with the issues of differentiation and autonomy by means of the realities of daily life, such as clothing, cologne, love—he receives from the father this new bit of information: "The shoes he's wearing are mine." At any moment in therapy, information that is related to the therapeutic goal immediately becomes relevant. The fact that Bill is wearing his father's shoes would not necessarily be useful, even though it brings instantly to mind the interesting tidbit of "walking in his father's footsteps." The therapist, however, who has a penchant for concrete metaphors, asks Bill to hand him a shoe. He has not yet formulated what he is going to do with that shoe, but as he examines it, he decides on a strategy that he will develop throughout the rest of the session.

Father: He doesn't have a pair of shoes to wear.

Minuchin (*looking at shoe*): What size are they?

Bill: We wear the same size—eleven.

Minuchin: Can I have the other one? (*Takes both shoes, wraps them in a paper, and gives them to father.*) I want you to take these shoes because these are your shoes.

Mother: You're going to have to buy a pair of shoes.

Minuchin (*to Bill*): Why do you wear your father's shoes?

Bill: Because—well—it's the same size as mine. Mine are worn out. It doesn't matter, because they are the same size.

Minuchin: How much money do you have in the bank?

Bill: About $4000.

Minuchin: Four thousand dollars. That is not much, because a pair of shoes like this must cost $50.

Father: You're wrong. I paid $14 for those at a wholesale house, honest to God, I swear.

Minuchin (*to Bill*): But when you go to buy a pair of shoes, you will buy a pair of shoes that cost $50 for yourself. You will buy a pair of shoes that are your size and that will cost $50. You can buy them for more, but it shouldn't be less. And I want *you* to do it. I am very, very concerned because you will not know where your skin finishes until you begin to find what is immediately next to your skin. I want to teach you where you are, and I want to begin by teaching you who you are. Then, we will begin by very simple things, like the things that are close to your body. I want you to go and buy yourself a pair of shoes. Do you know how to buy clothing?

The therapist uses the shoes as a concrete vehicle for dealing with issues of differentiation, building on common sense knowledge: "Wearing your father's shoes is confusing," "Your skin is a container of yourself," "You cannot know where you are if you don't know who you are." "Everybody knows" that these are objective realities. Out of these universal truths the therapist fashions a task that requires the identified patient to become involved in activities with the extrafamilial.

Bill: Just walk in and buy it?

Minuchin: Have you bought clothing for yourself, or are you a person who always buys the same kind of thing?

Bill: I don't normally buy too much. I buy the same things.

Minuchin: Let's find out from Rob. (*To Rob.*) Do you know how to select for yourself?

Rob: Yeah.

Minuchin: You will accompany Bill, but you will not do anything before Bill tells you. (*To Bill.*) If you like a pair of shoes and you want an opinion, then you can ask Rob and Rob will say yes or no. But don't ask him before you have decided. Okay?

Bill: Okay.

Minuchin: You will buy yourself—how many shirts do you have?

Bill: I have about seven shirts—six or seven shirts.

Minuchin: But you like this one more? (*The patient is also wearing the father's shirt.*) Why?

Bill: I don't like it any more or any less than the others.

Minuchin: But you need a couple of shirts more?

Bill: Yes, I can always use shirts, I guess. But I can use my father's.

Minuchin: No, no, no, no, because then you don't know who you are. I want you to begin to know what your body is by buying things that are yours. I want you and Rob to select a store where you will buy yourself some clothes. I don't want you to use your father's things. This is very

confusing. If you are going to know where you are, you start by knowing first what is your body. You start to know your body by beginning to clothe it. Okay? I don't know if you are yourself or you are your father, if you are in your father's shoes.
Bill: Okay.

The therapist constructs out of a pair of borrowed shoes a universal symbol of the meaning of individuation which he then uses to increase the separation between the father and son, to support the sibling holon, and to facilitate the re-entry of the identified patient into the extrafamilial context. The construction of the task has concrete elements: the identified patient is instructed to buy four shirts, two pairs of pants, and a dozen pairs of socks besides the pair of shoes. He leaves the office barefooted while his father carries the wrapped shoes. All of these elements contribute to an intensity to the therapist's construction.

Therapy continues for eight months. The identified patient is never hospitalized, although he has moments of disorganizing panic and suicidal ideation for over four months. A follow-up five years later shows the family members functioning well. The identified patient has moved away from the family and works independently, the younger brother works in the father's business, and the parents maintain clear, autonomous boundaries.

FAMILY TRUTHS

The therapist pays attention to the family's justifications of their transactions and uses their same worldview to expand their functioning. This is a kind of aikido, in which the therapist uses the family's own momentum to initiate a different direction: "Because you are concerned parents, you will give your child space to grow." "You will not rob him of his voice." "You will cut their wires." "You will demand respect." "You will show respect." "You will let her fail." Once the therapist has selected from the family's own culture the metaphors that symbolize their narrowed reality, he uses them as a construction whenever they appear or can be introduced, transforming them into a label that points up the family reality and suggests the direction of change. "Ah-ha, tightening the wires again!" This metaphor heightens the experience of the undesirable restraint. This technique corresponds to the second level of Berger and Luckmann's topology, rearranging simple explanatory schemas.

In the Scott family, the family reality is that the 17-year-old son John is truanting and shoplifting, regardless of the family's help or any punishment they have imposed. They feel he must be psychologically warped, because no normal child would continue shoplifting after he has been punished by being deprived of his hi-fi and motorcycle. The dysfunctional structure of this family is that the mother and children—John and his younger brother—form a holon which excludes the father, a guidance counselor.

In the therapeutic construction, the family's framing of the son is narrowed down to two unacceptable alternatives. Either the child is delinquent, or if he's not aware of his actions, he is crazy. When the mother refuses to accept either alternative, the therapist suggests another possibility: seek out the father's view of the situation. Within this construction there is a possibility for change in the family structure, strengthening the father's position in the executive holon. Ten minutes into the first session, the mother, John, and his brother have been explaining the psychological makeup of the identified patient as a justification for his behavior.

Minuchin (to mother): Let me ask you, do you think John is crazy?

Mother: Do I think he's crazy! No.

Minuchin: Do you think he knows what he does?

Mother: If you had asked me this when we first started in December, I would have said yes. He's cutting because he's a normal boy who wants to get out of class; there are other things that interest him. Once we started taking away these things that are so precious to him, then this is where I got concerned.

Minuchin: Then, you think he's crazy.

Mother: What do you mean by crazy?

Minuchin: I assume it is a person who does certain things and who is unaware that he's doing these things.

Mother: Well, he's aware that he's doing them, but he's not aware of why.

Minuchin: Do you think that he has weird behavior?

Father: My wife objected when I used the term "abnormal."

Minuchin: Maybe you think he's delinquent?

Mother: Delinquent? No. No, because this boy at home—

Minuchin (to father): Let me ask you, do you think he is a delinquent?

Father: In his behavior, yes.

Minuchin: That means, you think shoplifting is delinquent?

Father: Yes, it is, certainly.

Minuchin (to mother): But you don't think it is delinquent?

Mother: Well, when you say delinquent, I like to get an overall picture. Delinquent in certain things that he's done, yes; but as an overall boy with his home behavior and everything—

Minuchin: Don't you think that he knows that he shouldn't shoplift?

Mother: Certainly.

Minuchin: But, he's not delinquent?

Mother: He's delinquent in that he's doing it, but he knows he shouldn't.

Minuchin: There are two alternatives—either he's delinquent or he's crazy—

Mother (whispering): Delinquent or he's crazy?

Minuchin: Because if he does shoplifting, which he knows he should not do, and he's not a delinquent, it would appear that he's crazy.

The therapist, who has been very attentive to the family language, has been building confusion by accepting the mother's logical statements and carrying them to a pseudo-logical conclusion that is unacceptable. His intention is to weaken the certainty of the mother's control as a family reality and to introduce the father's reality as an alternative that is worth consideration.

Mother: Well, if you want me to make a choice, then I'll have to say he's delinquent. He's done something wrong.

Minuchin: You prefer delinquency?

Mother: Yes. He has done something which I think he knows was wrong.

Minuchin (to both parents): I think you need to make up your mind because then you will be effective. (*To mother.*) I think that you are copping out by saying that John is sick. I think you are ineffective.

Mother: We're not saying he was sick. We were told—

Minuchin: And you don't believe that.

Mother: I don't. No, that's why we're here. I didn't come to this conclusion.

Minuchin: I think you're helping John.

Mother: I'm a protective mother. I'll agree with you there.

Minuchin: I think you are helping John to be delinquent.

Mother: Well, please, will you tell me how to stop?

The wife is ready to shed her constructions but retain control of the parental functions by accepting the therapist's view. For the therapist to give her advice would maintain her monopoly on parenting while she was seeming to embrace an alternative. The therapist chooses instead to develop and support a pluralistic worldview, one that includes a dialectic interchange between the parents.

Minuchin: I think that your husband could.
Mother: You think he could—
Minuchin: Did you ask him?
Mother: Uh, ask him what? To help me? I wasn't aware—no.
Minuchin (to John, who is seated between parents): Now, move out. (*To husband.*) Sit near your wife, and maybe you can talk with her about how you can help her so that she does not have John continue doing weird and delinquent things. That's what this kid is doing. He's doing delinquent things.
Mother: I agree with you there. I said that he was delinquent, but—

The wife tries to maintain control by agreeing with the therapist and insisting on her dialog with him.

Minuchin: Talk with your husband, because I think he has a lot of clear ideas. You have very fuzzy ideas, and I think he can help you.

The therapist supports the spouse holon while lending weight to the husband's constructs.

Mother (to husband): Okay, I need help then, huh?
Father: We have different views on things, as I told you before, relating to this behavior. You know, his cutting school, skipping classes, puts him in a class of people that don't care what happens to them or to their lives. Now, I view this as parents who don't care themselves to see that their kids do the right things.

As the session continues, the therapist continues to support the father's view as a relevant alternative to the mother's now shaken certainty. This rearrangement of family facts facilitates a shift, in which a more flexible reality can be supported.

EXPERT ADVICE

With this technique the therapist presents a different explanation of the family reality, based on his own experience, knowledge, or wisdom: "I have seen other cases that . . ." "If you explore this area, you will find that . . ." The therapist may also shift explanatory positions, taking advantage of his stance as system leader to encompass a different family member's perspective or move to a different family perspective. From this position he can interpret the reality of the different family members, supporting deviation as a right, not as a heresy. The prescriptions that the therapist working with paradoxes gives are frequently based on his position as the expert.

In the Mullins family, the family reality is that the mother, who divorced the father two years ago, began almost immediately having difficulties in controlling her two adolescent daughters. The identified patient is 15-year-old Alice, who is failing in school even though the school has provided her with a teaching assistant to help her with her school work. Kathy, the 14-year-old, has passing grades, but the mother is concerned about both daughters' lack of effort and concern. The mother's uncertainty about her own life has resulted in an overemphasis on the deficits in the family.

The dysfunctional structure is related to the family change in organization after the parents' divorce, which resulted in an overinvolved system. The mother does not work and has become essentially a children-watcher, increasing her parental control at a period in which the children request more autonomy.

The therapeutic construction is based on acknowledging the mother's concern about her daughter's underachievement and carrying this theme forward to the point that people need to know their own effective level of functioning. Only by trying unaided, and possibly failing, will Alice find her areas of competence. She needs to own her own failure. This construction supports both mother and daughter's realities and acts as a boundary between them.

Minuchin: What is the problem? You will need to tell me, and convince me really, that there is a problem, so that I can help.

Mother: Well, I see the problem with both girls—and much more so with Alice—as the fact that they're not taking responsibility for themselves as far as their school work is concerned, and also their attitude, their goal in life. As far as Alice is concerned, she's frightened and she's negative and—

Alice: I can't help it.

Minuchin: So, that's your opinion of what's the trouble. Alice, I would like your opinion, and since your mother includes you, Kathy, I would like your opinion also. You know, I don't convince easily. Do you agree with what your mother said, Alice?

The mother presents the family's orientation toward pathology and helplessness; the therapist counters with a doubt that puts the responsibility of proof on the family. This gives him the power to select the family facts that are therapeutically relevant.

Alice: No. She's saying that she gets all upset because Kathy and I don't know what our goals in life are and our attitude toward school. She can't be convinced that I'm doing okay in school. You tell her and she doesn't believe you and she stays on your back.

Minuchin: So, you are doing very well in school?

Alice: Not very well—I'm passing.

Minuchin: Okay. So, you don't see that there is a problem in school, and in relation to life you are waiting because you are young and don't need to decide yet. Is that the idea?

Alice: I guess.

Minuchin: And you cannot convince your mother that everything is okay. Why is she so upset?

Alice: That's what I'd like to know.

Minuchin: Can you find out why she's so upset then?

Alice (to mother): Why are you so upset?

Mother: I guess it is your attitude. I don't want to see you fail because you're a bright girl.

Alice: But you can't accept the fact that I'm doing all right in school. You just stick to what you think is right.

Mother: And you have so much potential!

The mother-daughter dialog provides a field for exploring the way in which the mother arranges the daughter's reality. The mother insists on highlighting the "relevant reality" that is, a reality of deficits.

Minuchin: Do you want me to tell you what I see?

Alice: Uh-huh.

Minuchin: I see you and your mom being hooked to each other as if you are a much younger person than 15, and your mother is feeling that you cannot make it without her because she thinks that you are lazy or afraid or incompetent. Now I think that this is your life, and I know many kids who do a minimum of effort and they pass. That's their choice, you know. And your mother cannot accept that.

Alice: That's how she is. She doesn't accept anything.

Minuchin: I think you should fail on your own.

Alice: I don't want to fail!

Minuchin: But, you see, they ensure that you don't need to make any efforts—

Alice: I do make efforts!

Minuchin: —not to fail. Your mom, and the school are not allowing you to fail on your own. I think you should fail and know that you have failed and learn what you need to do. (*To mother.*) Why don't you let her fail?

Alice: I'm not going to fail!

The therapist highlights the consequences of failure as a constructive possibility. There are a number of elements in this construction. One is that by exaggerating the nature of the mother-daughter dance and insisting on failure, the therapist activates resistance in the identified patient, who insists that she will not fail. But also, by emphasizing failure as an exploration of competence, he sends to the identified patient a message of acceptance of her unknown capabilities which contrasts with the mother's emphasis on and fear of deficits.

When the therapist explores the sibling holon, he finds that Kathy, like the mother, takes a helping position regarding Alice. He expands the focus to include Kathy as a helper, casting her as Alice's lawyer and translator, and then highlights complementarity by making Kathy's help a response to Alice's request for help.

Minuchin: Now Alice, not only your mother and teacher, but your sister also helps. You are just extraordinary! How did you manage to develop a world of helpers around you?

Alice: They all like me. They want to help me.

Minuchin: It can't be just luck. It must be that you are an expert in being incompetent.

Kathy: How can you be an expert at that?

Minuchin: I want you to observe what happened, Alice. I asked you a question, and Kathy answered.

Kathy: Alice talked first.

Minuchin: And now your sister is supporting you. I just want you to notice that.

Alice: I know, I know.
Minuchin: I think you are an expert in making people do your work.
Alice: No way!

The therapist maintains focus on the active part that Alice has in organizing her family's response, complementing the family members' control of Alice with Alice's control of them.

Minuchin (to mother): You have a younger daughter who is the older sister of your older daughter, and I don't think that anybody is giving Alice a chance. Alice, you function minimally at school, but this is because nobody lets you grow up.
Alice: My mother expects too much, and she doesn't know the inside of my head. She says that I can do this and I can't do this and maybe I can't.
Minuchin: Then you need to work more. But they will not let you. Maybe if you begin to do a little bit more work on your own, maybe you will find out that you are almost as bright as your younger sister.

There are two elements in this intervention: one is a challenge, the other a support. By suggesting that Alice's sibling may be more intelligent, the therapist provokes Alice to prove him wrong. And by suggesting that with more work she may prove everybody wrong, the therapist emphasizes Alice's strength.

In the Reynolds family, the family reality is that the parents, Vera and George, have two married children and a younger daughter, Martha, a 17-year-old anorectic who alternates starvation and food binges. The parents see themselves as concerned people, who have been successful with the older children and are trying their best with the identified patient. Martha spends a large part of her life monitoring the parents' nontalking and trying to meet the mother and father's need for companionship.

The dysfunctional structure has come about through the course of a long marriage in which the parents have evolved a way of detouring conflicts through Martha. There are no dyadic holons that are not transformed into triads.

The therapeutic construction is to change the meaning of the symptom by rearranging the relationship among family members on the basis of the therapist's expertise. If the meaning of things is given by "the shadow that the universe casts on them," putting the symptom in a different universe will change its meaning.[2] The therapist uses this formulation as the basis for creating transactional pathways that will separate the child from the spouse holon.

Minuchin (to mother): What do you do?
Mother: I work for the city.
Minuchin: That means it's a nine-to-five job?
Mother: Yes.
Minuchin: Do you have any help?
Mother: No. I never did. Recently my husband has been helping me.
Martha: Mom, that's a lie and you know that. I've always helped you. I've done the dishes and vacuumed or washed the floor when I'm home on my summer vacation, and I put supper in the oven before you come home.
Mother: Martha, don't get all hyper now—
Martha: You said you had no help and that's what I—
Mother: Sometimes I did get help. When I asked for help, I got it, Martha.
Martha: Other times you didn't ask and I helped.
Father: Martha was helping quite a bit.
Mother: Okay, she was. She was making supper sometimes. But don't say it like she did it routinely every night. She did not.
Father: For a while there, it was pretty routine.
Martha: It was.

The nature of the triadic arrangement is such that when the mother and daughter reach a certain level of stress, the father is activated and takes the daughter's side. The therapist does not yet know if this is the preferred dance or just a movement in a larger dance in which a third member is activated whenever the other two enter into conflict.

Mother: It was. Right until she started getting real bad.
Minuchin: Vera, do you find that George and Martha sometimes team up and put you down? Martha, just now, got kind of hepped and kicked you.
Mother: I don't care. She does that a lot.
Minuchin: And then what happened with George?
Mother: He came to her rescue.
Father: Did I?
Minuchin: Yes, you did here. Absolutely you did. He does this at home?

Mother: He does that at home now that you mention it. Yes. Because when I used to reprimand her and scold her, he would tell me to be quiet and to stop the noise and leave her alone. He always came to her defense.

Father: That works both ways, too. Sometimes I would also tell Martha not to bother Mother at certain times of the day. I'm just trying to keep a happy medium. I'm sitting in the background. I'm just watching.

Clearly the father can dance with different partners without changing his steps. But by highlighting certain facts, the therapist focuses the view of family members on the patterned nature of their transaction.

Minuchin: Vera says that she experiences you being more in Martha's corner than in hers. (*To Martha.*) Are you very frail? I saw you taking Mom out very easily. You were not afraid of taking her on. You didn't need his help.

Martha: No.

Minuchin: No. Does that happen frequently that Dad feels that his weight will help you if you are in an argument with Mother? Will he try to make peace by joining with you?

Martha: No, not really. He'll just tell me, like, "Simmer down and leave her alone," or "Why don't you stop bothering her, let her do what she wants," or whatever, and then I feel guilty because my mother gets hurt in the situation, and I don't want anybody to be hurt.

The therapist starts with an automatic transaction in the family, a casual conversation. By framing it as an issue of taking sides in a quarrel, he makes the issues of autonomy, power, coalition, and guilt magically apparent in the family transaction.

Father: Don't get the wrong impression there. You've got the impression that I'm always doing this. No. Very seldom do I speak up.

Martha: But when he does, that's how it works.

Father: I don't want to see two people arguing foolishly. It's a foolish argument. If I'm sitting in one room and I hear an argument going on in the kitchen and I feel it's foolish—one will say one thing, another one will say another thing—it's nothing constructive, it's foolish—and they're both getting hot under the collar about it, naturally I'll step in.

Minuchin: So, you are a referee?
Father: You might call it that.

In this family of conflict avoiders, the therapist frames the father's function as a monitor of conflict.

Minuchin (to mother): Why would he do a thing like that? Do you get hurt easily?
Mother: I used to. I've got a shell on me now.
Father: We have a pillar of fire here (*pointing to wife*) and we have a pillar of fire here (*pointing to daughter*). We have two positives. They are very outspoken, both of them.
Minuchin: George, is it necessary to monitor their fights?
Father: No, it's not necessary, but I feel I should step in before somebody says something they will be sorry for later on.
Minuchin: You don't like a fight in your family?
Father: No, I don't.
Minuchin: What about between you and Vera?
Mother: We don't talk.
Father: If I feel a fight coming on, my wife gets excited or I get excited—but she'll get excited more than me, and then she'll get excited more and more up to a point where I feel I better stop—I just get up and either walk out of the house or walk into another room just to stop it.
Minuchin: And that works?
Father: It works, but then she's mad at me for a couple of days. She won't talk to me.
Mother: We've gone where you don't talk to me for a month and I give you the same treatment.
Minuchin (to Martha): What do you do then?
Martha (laughing): Well, I withdraw into my own world. It's more safe and secure there.
Minuchin: That means then Mom is in her corner, Dad is in his corner, and you go into your corner? Great family! How do you get out of it? Don't you try to talk with Mom or with Dad or try to patch it up?
Martha: Sure, I try to, but it is very uncomfortable. They're not talking with each other, and then I feel I've done something because my mother, without realizing it, accidentally might snap at me for something. I figure what did I do and I just better keep quiet, and I'll just go in my own world and not have to worry about getting rejected again by them—by their snapping at me.

Father: Martha, I don't snap at you.

Martha: No, Mom does though. But my father will always talk to me, though. It's like, "Well, if your mother doesn't want to talk, that's fine." He'll just say something like that. But then I feel guilty, because I should be doing something. I'm living in the same house and I should be making them have a more pleasant life. You know, I have to make them talk and enjoy their life.

Minuchin: And are you successful?

Martha: No. So I punish myself for this and go on a binge.

Minuchin: Then is that helpful?

Martha: Well, to me it is. It just temporarily relieves the problems. It's like alcohol or drugs. It doesn't solve anything.

Minuchin: So, I see here two therapists already—Father, who when you are fighting with Mom, tries to put oil on rough waters, and you, who try to monitor and help these people. And you are not a very good therapist. You are not very successful.

After labeling the father a referee, the therapist highlights the daughter's symptom as serving a similar function, but he adds an image of her as a healer.

Martha: I can't be. They won't let me. They say, "Mind your own business."

Mother: It's none of your business what goes on between us.

Martha: That, to me, is a rejection, because I feel I'm part of the family. I should be doing something.

Minuchin: How long have you been trying to cure them?

Martha: I never thought about it. Now that I think about it, it's about the time the anorexia started.

The identified patient accepts the therapeutic construction and locates it in time. The symptom acquires a different meaning: instead of being an individual illness, it becomes a family cure.

Minuchin: That means for four or five years you have been trying to cure them?

Martha: Yeah.

Minuchin: Oh, my girl, you need better techniques than the ones that you have. In four or five years, you should have changed them. (*To parents.*) She tries to heal you. She tries to bring happiness to you, and she's just not good at that. (*To daughter.*) Have you ever tried to get some training in how to increase harmony and happiness?

In a light mood, the therapist suggests a possible alternative for the symptom bearer, to shed her ineffective binges and become an effective problem solver.

Martha: No. The only thing I would ever do is ask them, "Why aren't you talking?" "It's none of your business." Then I feel that they're uncomfortable by my trying to do anything. So I wasn't even much thinking of myself as a therapist before, but now I think I can help this family.

Minuchin: Maybe not a therapist, but a healer. Somebody who tries to bring harmony and happiness in a family. I would like you, Martha, to talk with your parents about the ways in which they frustrate your attempts to help them.

The therapist uses the construction of the girl as a healer to change the nature of the family relationship, transforming the passive position of binger into an active interpersonal task. The identified patient is put in charge of her parents, with the goal of prompting them to reject this increased intrusion.

Martha (to parents): How am I going to say this so it makes sense, so you can understand it? It's like I have to go on a guilt trip because you aren't talking. You're my parents and I love you, but if you don't love each other, I feel guilty, and I can't live my life unless I know you're happy. You see, you try to hide it. Like you say it's your own business, but still it isn't your business because I live in the same house and I have to see this. It's not the fighting, it's the not talking that bothers me.

Mother: We don't get into arguments that way.

Martha: Well, see how it's affected me? I see you don't talk to people, so I go to school and I figure, subconsciously, I can't talk to people. I don't know how to, you know. If I heard you having a conflict and resolving it, then I could learn from that, you know.

Mother: But, Martha, it's taken us thirty years to arrive at this attitude that we have—thirty-three years.

Martha: But the thing is I can't be happy unless I know you're happy.

Mother: But I'm happy in my little world and your father's happy in his little world.

Parents: And you should be happy in your little world.

Martha: Do you think it could be better? I know you don't want it to be better, but could it be?

Minuchin: You see, it's a very interesting thing what Martha is saying. She is saying that you really need her very badly because you, together, cannot hack it.

Martha: I feel that I'm bringing you happiness in some way, you know.

Minuchin: I don't think your parents understand you. I don't think that they understood what you just said.

Martha: Neither do I.

Minuchin: I don't think that they are hearing you. You are saying something very simple. You are saying that unless you can help them, they cannot make it.

The therapist has been egging the identified patient on to continue her job as her parents' healer for over fifteen minutes. In the process, the identified patient addresses herself to the parents as a couple, instead of pursuing her usual negotiation with each of them separately. The parents respond—sometimes annoyed, at times placating—as a holon. The therapeutic construction's exaggeration is intended to produce the parents' rejection of the girl's help and to create distance from her.

Minuchin: Talk with Dad and talk with Mom.

Martha: It's things like—you guys figure that's your life and I should just stay out of it. Is that how you feel? Is that what you're trying to tell me?

Mother: Um-hum.

Martha: I don't understand it. None of it makes any sense.

Minuchin: You see, my feeling is, Martha, that your parents know that they need you. You couldn't have such a strong feeling toward helping them unless they are telling you—

Martha: That they want it.

Minuchin: That they want it. How does your mother tell you that she likes you to help? They must be doing it in some way. I don't know that they know how they do it, but they must be doing it. They must be telling you in some way. How do they do it?

The therapist changes the locus of control of the girl's life. She is now framed as responding to parental control. This is a radical shift from the previous focus on the identified patient as a doer, and it has the purpose of activating the identified patient to distance herself from her parents.

Minuchin: Martha, you are really an exploited little girl. You are pretty, you are seventeen, and you don't have a boy friend. Do you have many girl friends?

Martha: No, I won't be close to anybody. I'm too afraid. I can't do that.

Father: You had a close girl friend once.

Martha: Who? No, I'm not close to her. No.

Father: That's your closest girl friend, though.

Mother: She was your closest girl friend.

Father: You went on vacations together—

Minuchin (to parents): Hold it a moment.

Martha: How do they know I'm close to her? How can they say that? How can they say that?

Minuchin: That is one of the ways in which they pull you. Just now, you were telling me something about your life and then—

Martha: They think they know about it.

Minuchin: They entered and they are pulling you. You see, I am concerned that you will never, never leave your home.

The therapist uses a simple family transaction to support his construction of strong parental control.

Minuchin (to mother): How old are you?

Mother: Fifty-four.

Minuchin: Fifty-four. So probably you have what—25 more years of life?

Mother: If I'm lucky.

Minuchin: If you are going to 80. And how old are you, George?

Father: Fifty-four.

Minuchin: Okay. So, maybe—how old are you, Martha? Seventeen. They will die around 80, so you have 25 years to remain at home. So, 25 and 17—you will be a very immature, 42-year-old single woman when you are ready to leave home.

Martha: No, I don't want that to happen.

The therapist projects a dark future with a bleak prognosis in order to provoke resistance and increase the identified patient's distance from her parents.

Minuchin: I think that that will happen, because they are busy asking you to help them to become happier. And you are spending all of your time looking at your dad and your mom. You look so much at them that you don't have time to look elsewhere. Why don't you have a boy friend?

Martha: I'm too afraid. I don't want to go out of the house.

Minuchin: Oh, that is—that means—you are saying that you are using them also? They are using you and you are using them?

Martha: Yeah, this one kid keeps calling me, and I tell my father to tell him I'm not home. And he does; he says, "Oh, you just missed her. She just walked out the door."

Minuchin: That means you use them to defend yourself against the world outside.

Martha (laughing): These are my weapons.

Minuchin: You are a very interesting family. It's very, very interesting, because clearly she uses you also. I thought that you used her, but she uses you.

The therapist moves back to the parents and challenges them for allowing the identified patient to exploit them and use them to avoid facing the world outside. During the rest of the session, which lasts three hours, the therapist shifts the focus, periodically highlighting the different uses that the family members make of each other. But in all of his constructions he keeps legitimizing a structure that distances the parents from the child and supports differentiation.

In addressing himself to a family's worldview, the therapist works from a distant position. He introduces concepts that challenge concepts. Theoretically, the idea itself is the intervention, for in accommodating to the new conceptualization, the family enters a period of confusion, crisis, and readjustment. The process is like dropping a stone into a pond: a ripple effect results, which has nothing to do with the nature of the stone or the agent who dropped it.

But in life, the idea is not separate from the therapist who introduces it. Separating the two is an artificial construct, which has the danger of emphasizing the idea, shutting off the view of the interpersonal context in which it occurs. Some schools of family therapy that regard cognitive challenge as the major level for therapeutic change have tried to keep the introduction of a challenging conceptual schema pure of the impact of the therapists themselves. But they have now shifted their position, recognizing the participation of the therapist as the challenger.

Convincing the family of a new concept requires the therapist's partic-ipation. Furthermore, the separation of a cognitive challenge from a structural challenge is an artificial construct. A challenge to the family worldview is simultaneously a challenge to its interactional structure, just as a challenge to its structure is a challenge to its worldview. Cogni-tive challenge simply does not exist in isolation. With this caveat firmly in mind, however, the therapist can make effective use of cognitive schemas.

16 Paradoxes

By Peggy Papp

The Ackerman Brief Therapy Project was organized in 1974 under my and Olga Silverstein's direction to experiment with the use of paradox in treating families with symptomatic children. Initially it was composed of eight self-selected family therapists previously trained at the Ackerman Institute for Family Therapy. Building on the ideas of others who have made use of paradox in family therapy, such as Jay Haley, Milton Erickson, Mara Selvini-Palazzoli, Paul Watzlawick, John Weakland, and Richard Fisch, the project quickly took a direction of its own and developed its own unique characteristics.

Our use of paradox is based on an understanding of three concepts: the concept of the family as a self-regulatory system, the concept of the symptom as a mechanism for self-regulation, and the concept of systemic resistance to change, resulting from the preceding two. Because the symptom is used to regulate a dysfunctional part of the system, if the symptom is eliminated, that part of the system will be left unregulated.

The most common example of this is parents who divert their conflict through a child's activating a symptom. In alleviating the symptom in the child, the therapist allows the unresolved issues between the parents to become exposed, creating a great deal of anxiety and a strong resistance to change. We use paradox primarily as a clinical tool for dealing with this resistance and circumventing a power struggle between the family and the therapist.

Families with symptomatic children usually present the therapist with a contradictory request, asking that the symptom be changed without changing their system. The therapist deals with this contradiction through a series of drastic redefinitions that connect the symptom with the system in such a way that one cannot be changed without changing the other. In so doing, the therapist sets the terms for the therapeutic contest. The central issue is no longer how to eliminate the symptom but what will happen if it is eliminated; the therapeutic argument is shifted from the "problem"—who has it, what caused it, and how do you get rid of it—to how the family will survive without it, who will be affected by its absence, in what way, and what will they do about it.

Through this systemic redefining, a perceptual crisis is created. Following it, the family finds it increasingly difficult to regulate itself through a symptom and begins to regulate itself differently.

One of the distinguishing features of our work is the differential and alternate use of paradox with other types of interventions. Experience has shown that paradox is neither always necessary nor always desirable. Our criterion for its use is based on our evaluation of the degree of resistance to change in that part of the system that the symptom is regulating. We test this resistance through a number of trial runs, and if it is responsive to direct interventions, there is no need to resort to the use of paradox. Also there are certain crisis situations, such as violence, sudden grief, attempted suicide, loss of employment, or unwanted pregnancy, in which a paradox would be inappropriate, as the therapist needs to move in quickly to provide structure and control. We reserve paradoxical interventions for those covert, long-standing, repetitious patterns of interaction that do not respond to direct interventions such as logical explanations or rational suggestions.

Interventions may be classified as direct or compliance-based, referring to the therapist's expectation that the family will comply with them, and as paradoxical or defiance-based, referring to the therapist's expectation that the family will defy them.[1]

DIRECT INTERVENTIONS, COMPLIANCE-BASED

By direct interventions are meant advice, explanations, suggestions, interpretations, and tasks that are meant to be taken literally and followed as prescribed. They are aimed at directly changing family rules or roles. They include coaching parents on how to control children, redistributing jobs among family members, establishing disciplinary rules, regulating privacy, establishing age hierarchy, and providing information that the family lacks. They also include promoting open communication, eliciting feelings, giving personal feedback to the family and interpreting family interaction. Direct interventions are given with the expectation that they will be followed and therefore are used when it is felt the family will respond to them.

PARADOXICAL INTERVENTIONS, DEFIANCE-BASED

A paradoxical intervention is one that, if followed, will accomplish the opposite of what it is seemingly intended to accomplish. It depends for success on the family's defying the therapist's instructions or following them to the point of absurdity and recoiling. If a family continually defies compliance-based interventions, it can be safely assumed there is some hidden interaction in the system that undermines their usefulness—some secret alliance, contest, or coalition that the family is reluctant to reveal or change. The target of the systemic paradox is this hidden interaction that expresses itself in a symptom. The three major techniques used in designing and applying a systemic paradox are: redefining, prescribing, and restraining.

The purpose of redefining is to change the family's perception of the problem. The symptom is redefined from a foreign element outside the system to an essential part of it. Behavior that maintains the symptom is defined as benignly motivated to preserve family stability. Anger is defined as caring, suffering as self-sacrifice, distancing as a way of reinforcing closeness, and so on. Rather than trying to change the system directly, the therapist supports it, respecting the inner emotional logic on which it runs.

Having been defined positively, the symptom-producing cycle of interaction is then prescribed as an inevitable conclusion of the family's own logic. When the cycle that produced the symptom is consciously enacted, it loses its power to produce a symptom. The secret rules of the game are made explicit and the family must take responsibility for its own actions. In the words of Michael Foucault, the family "is led through a state in which it is confronted by itself and forced to argue against the demands of its own truth."[2]

A prerequisite for prescribing this cycle is an accurate knowledge of the relation between the symptom and the system and the manner in which they activate one another.

If the therapist is to be consistent with the above two steps, whenever the family shows signs of changing, she must restrain them. If indeed the symptom is an essential element in the functioning of this system, and the therapist respects that system, she can only worry about change. As the family recoils from this prescription and presses for change, the therapist regulates its pace. She constantly enumerates the consequences of the change and anticipates the new difficulties that will arise, predicts how they will affect the system, and cautiously allows the family to change in spite of these.

A systemic paradox is used in the treatment of the Allen family, in which an eight-year-old boy is failing in school. The therapist determines that the symptom serves the function of keeping the mother's disappointment focused on her son, Billy, rather than on her husband. The husband is failing in business and, rather than redoubling his efforts, is sinking into apathy, leaving the mother to shoulder much of the financial burden. He gives off signals that he would collapse if confronted openly with this issue, and the mother collaborates in protecting him. Whenever she becomes angry at his lack of ambition, she nags Billy to straighten out and make something of himself, do his homework, practice his violin, or clean up his room. The mother and Billy end up fighting, and the father retires to the den to watch television. Both parents deny there is a marital problem, the wife stating, "My husband doesn't like to fight, and I've accepted this."

The therapist tells the mother it is important for her to continue to express her disappointment in Billy, because otherwise she might begin to express her dissatisfaction with her husband. This would be risky, as her husband might become depressed, and since Billy is younger and more resilient than her husband, he can take it better. Billy is advised to continue to protect his father by keeping the mother's disappointment focused on him, and the father is commended for his cooperation. The mother has an immediate recoil, saying, "You're suggesting I fight with my eight-year-old son instead of my husband, a grown man? Why should I damage my son to protect my husband?" thus defining her own predicament. The husband supports the therapist, saying he thinks her suggestion is a good one "because Billy bounces right back. With him it doesn't last for a long period of time, and he doesn't get depressed as I do. Besides, we can't know for sure if it's doing him any damage." The mother is outraged at her husband's validation of the therapist's perception and proceeds to fight with him. The conflict is refocused onto the parents, and Billy is released from his middle position. Defining and prescribing their system in a way that is both accurate and unacceptable makes it impossible for them to continue it.

Several mistakes can be made in trying to follow this procedure. The most common one is simply prescribing the symptom without connecting it with the system, "Billy, you should keep failing in school and disappointing Mother." This lacks therapeutic impact, which depends on redefining the symptom as serving the system, connoting both positively, and prescribing both.

Another common error is merely prescribing the system, as in "Billy, you should continue to fail in school and disappoint Mother; Mother, you should continue to fight with Billy; and Father, you should continue to withdraw." Again, the system is not connected with the symptom in a circular definition.

REVERSALS, DEFIANCE-COMPLIANCE-BASED

A reversal is an intervention in which the therapist directs someone in the family to reverse her attitude or behavior around a crucial issue in the hope that it will elicit a paradoxical response from another family member. It is both defiance and compliance-based. It requires the conscious cooperation of the family member who is being instructed by the therapist and the defiance of the family member who is receiving the results of the instruction. Reversals are useful when one member of the family is cooperative and will follow direct advice and another will resist it. For example, in the Gordon family, in which the wife resents an overly close relationship between her husband and his mother, the therapist instructs the wife privately to reverse her attitude regarding the relationship. Rather than taking her usual stance of opposing it, which only solidifies it, she should, the therapist suggests, find ways of praising the beauty of this rare mother-son devotion and should encourage her husband to spend even more time with his mother. The wife, as expected, complies with the therapist's instructions; the husband, as expected, defies his wife's instructions by becoming less involved with his mother.

Reversals can be used effectively in helping parents handle rebellious children. Remarkable results can be achieved in a short period of time if the parents are willing to follow the therapist's coaching. When reversals are given, the person who is on the receiving end should not be present, as the success of a reversal depends on that person being surprised and reacting spontaneously to an unexpected change of attitude. For example, in the Draper family, with a 13-year-old son who is flunking school as a reaction to the constant pressuring of his parents, the parents are instructed to tell the youngster that they are really not that concerned about his grades because if he has to stay home and attend summer school, at least they will know he is safe and they will be able to keep their eye on him all summer.

Reversals are used when it is felt one segment of the family is capable of reversing a core position that will affect another segment of the family. A combination of these techniques is used with most families during the course of treatment, based on the therapist's evaluation of the compliance-defiance factor.

CONSULTATION GROUP AS A GREEK CHORUS

Another distinguishing feature of our work is the use of a consultation group to underline the therapist's interventions. This group is composed of colleagues who alternate in observing one another from behind the one way mirror. This group acts as a Greek chorus, providing a running commentary on the interaction between the family and the therapist. It is the voice of the family prophet, proclaiming the systemic truths in the family and predicting the future course of events. Its major preoccupation is with the phenomenon of systemic change. Regular messages are sent in from the group commenting on this phenomenon, how it will come about, what the consequences will be, who will be affected by them, in what way, and what the alternatives are.

The messages are formed in collaboration with the therapist, who has the final say as to their content and decides on what position to take in relation to them. At the therapist's discretion, the group can be used to support, confront, confuse, challenge, or provoke the family, with the therapist free to agree with them or oppose them.

The group is presented to the family in a way that invests it with the highest possible authority. The family are told that they are privileged to have this special resource available to them, that the group is composed of experts in the field who are authorities on their particular kind of problem. If the family so desire, they are introduced to the group, but have no further contact with it. It remains at a distance, an invisible eye, an anonymous voice, lending the impact of objectivity.

The group may be used in the following ways. We believe, however, that we have only begun to explore its potential.

The group is sometimes used simply to praise or support certain aspects of the family that need strengthening. For example, in the Collins family, in which the husband presents a gruff exterior to cover a tender heart, his wife often fails to appreciate his tenderness, as it is expressed through gestures rather than words. Her lack of appreciation discourages him from making further advances, and he retreats behind his "don't give a damn" pose. When he gives her a book of her favorite poems for her birthday, the group uses the occasion to define him as a romantic figure, sending in the message: "The women in the group were touched by Tom's beautiful gift to Myrna. They wish their husbands would think of things like that. They have always felt there was a romantic side to Tom, and they are curious as to how it will express itself in the future. They are taking bets on it but won't reveal them."

In the Blake family, the group sends in a message supporting the husband's right to make his own decision as to whether he will attend the therapy sessions. He refused to come to the first two sessions as a reaction to his wife's persistent coercion, and when he did agree to come for only one session, she used that session to berate him for his lack of concern for his family: "You wouldn't give a damn if we were all dying." The consultation team counters the mother's pressure: "The group, not having met Jim before, is impressed with his ability to take care of himself. Somehow the family mythology had led us to believe differently. Therefore, we respect his decision to come to terms with his life in his own way and feel sure his wife will do the same." Thus supported, he begins coming to the sessions regularly.

At other times the group is used as a public opinion poll, to take odds on the course of change. As the sessions progress, the opinion of the group may shift, depending upon which way they wish to throw their weight. In the Richards family, in which the therapist is trying to get the parents to keep the children out of their marital issues, the therapist begins the interview by stating that the group is split on the crucial issue of whether the parents will be able to prevent the children from sabotaging their new-kindled romance. Half the group believes the children will win, but the other half are rooting for the parents. As the session continues and the parents begin to lose, the count shifts, and the therapist informs the family that according to the latest poll, all but one person in the group believe the parents have lost the battle. That one person is holding out, because he believes that the father is stronger than all three children and will find a way of regaining ground.

There are many different ways of splitting the opinion of the group in order to make a therapeutic point. Sometimes it is divided along sex lines to increase the incentive of each partner in the battle of the sexes: "All the women in the group predict it will be the husband who will be responsible for creating the next crisis by drinking too much, but all the men believe the wife will do it by involving her mother in their private affairs."

In families in which women's liberation is a hot issue, the opinion poll of the group is used as a spur for disentanglement. A mirror image of the conflicting issues is constructed in the group and fed back to the family.

In the Palmer family, the mother is ambivalent over her own liberation, alternating between an obsessive involvement in a triangle with her husband and son and a concerted effort to get a doctorate in anthropology. The group defines and exaggerates the conflict: "Mother's predicament has created a political division among the women in the group. One-third feel she should stay home and devote her entire time and attention to her husband and son, as this is the highest achievement a woman can aspire to; one-third feel she has already done this for fifteen years with little appreciation from either husband or son for her efforts and now she has the right to fulfill her own creativity and potential; the remaining third agree with the latter, that mother has the right to fulfill her own potential, but is worried that father and son may become totally helpless without her and she should therefore remain at home." Hearing the issues defined in these terms, the mother decides that only the second alternative is acceptable to her. She gets her doctorate and gives up trying to change father and son.

Since surprise and confusion are important elements of change, the group is also sometimes used to produce them. It may send in a message to arouse the family's curiosity, stir up their imagination, or provoke them into revealing hidden information. These messages are sometimes left deliberately unclear, as an invitation to the family to fill in the gaps.

In the Olsen family, the parents are extremely closed off and secretive, creating a stilted atmosphere of vague foreboding that is difficult to decipher. Their adolescent son, Micky, constantly provokes them with disruptive behavior in an effort to counteract the deadly atmosphere. This produces a round robin in which the parents engage in a never-ending battle to quiet their son and the son engages in a never-ending battle to disquiet the parents. The therapist and group speculate that some kind of well-guarded family secret is creating this foreboding atmosphere and the concomitant turmoil.

The therapist returns from a consultation with the group to deliver their message:

Papp: The group has the impression that this family is like a prison, but it's unclear who is the jailer and who are the prisoners. Somebody here secretly in his heart might want to escape, but this might be devastating to the family, as it is a very close family. (*Turns to the boy.*) In a sense, Micky, your job is to keep this game of prisoners and jailers going, as in reality that person might try to make a break for it.

Micky: I'm the one that's locked up.
Papp: I'm not so sure—are you being locked up or locking everyone else up?

During the next session the mother reveals she has been thinking of leaving the family for some time. Now that the issue is out in the open, it can be dealt with between the parents, and the boy's symptom subsides.

One of the most potent uses of the group is the creation of a therapeutic triangle resulting from an ongoing, planned conflict between the therapist and the group. In this triangle, the group usually takes the position of antagonist of change, and the therapist, who has the personal relationship with the family, takes the position of protagonist of change. The group regularly warns the therapist against the consequences of systemic change and continually defines the part of the system that is working against this. The therapist swings back and forth as family resistance shifts, alternately agreeing and disagreeing with the group.

In the Marble family, in which the symptom is the daughter's inability to leave home, the therapist might initially oppose the group by saying, "I disagree with the group that Linda needs to stay home to protect her mother from being alone with her father. I believe mother is capable of handling father and the two of them can manage on their own." If the parents disprove this, the therapist can shift to, "I see now what the group was trying to tell me about your difficulty in being alone with one another. I apologize for having misjudged the situation. It seems the group was right and for the time being Linda needs to remain at home to console her mother."

The therapeutic triangle created among the group, family, and therapist gives the therapist a unique maneuverability, emanating from a liberating distance. In *A Journey to Ixtlan*, the Indian philosopher, Don Juan, advises the author, Carlos Castenada, "If one wants to stop our fellow men, one must always be outside the circle that presses them. That way one can always direct the pressure." Carlos has asked Don Juan's advice about a friend of his who cannot control his unruly son. Don Juan suggests that the father go to Skid Row, hire a frightening derelict, instruct the derelict to follow him and his son, and in response to a prearranged cue, after some objectional behavior on his son's part, leap from the hiding place, pick up the child, and spank the living daylights out of him. The father must then console his son and help him regain his confidence. This should be repeated several times in different places. Don Juan assures Carlos that "the boy would soon change his view of the world."[4]

The consultation group serves a function similar to the derelict, as an agent "outside the world that presses them." And the therapist is in a similar position to the father, who "directs the pressure."

The physical procedure for using the group can be structured in a variety of ways. Our regular procedure is for the therapist to excuse herself near the end of the session to consult with the group in a different room, leaving the video camera running to record the family interaction. The therapist then returns with a communication that is usually written and read aloud to the family with a proper solemnity. A copy of this communication is then mailed to all family members so they can study it at their convenience. This lends an additional importance and authority to the message. After reading the communication, the therapist terminates the session, not allowing the family to dissipate the content through an intellectual discussion of it. It is dropped like a time bomb and left to explode at a later date as the family comprehends it.

The group is free to interrupt at any time during the session or call the therapist out to make suggestions. A prearranged signal may be agreed upon by the group and therapist, by which the group interrupts at a particular point in time with a particular message. If cotherapy is used, a three-way strategy is worked out between the two therapists and the group.

The question is often asked on this subject, "What does one do if one doesn't have a group?" The same principles may be applied by a regular cotherapy team, with each therapist taking an opposing position on various issues. Or a trainee and supervisor may agree on a division of opinion around a central theme. Or even a single therapist may change her own opinion: "I've been thinking about your family a lot, and I realize I've been making a serious mistake in trying to get mother and Suzie to stop fighting, because that's the only time father becomes involved in the family, and if they stopped, father might totally disappear. So for the time being, Suzie, it's important for you to fight with your mother until she can find another way to keep father at home."

Another question that is raised concerns the effect this has on the child. "Isn't it harmful to tell the child to continue destructive behavior in order to save the parents?" We believe that is what the child is actually doing, and by making the covert overt, we are releasing her from that position, at the same time making the parents aware of it.

FOLLOWING THROUGH ON A SYSTEMIC PARADOX

After the systemic paradox has been formulated and delivered comes the difficult task of following through on it. During the next session the family will most likely not mention the message. They have many ingenious methods for trying to wipe it out, including ignoring it, forgetting it, dismissing it, contradicting it, or coming in with a new crisis that has nothing to do with the original problem. The next step requires the therapist assiduously to hold on to her circular definition of the problem and continually to fit family behavior into the new framework. That requires the conviction on the part of the therapist that her perception is accurate. Beginners often have difficulty delivering a paradoxical message as they lack this conviction. Afraid the message may sound absurd, they become self-conscious and deliver it in a tentative way which makes the family feel they are being facetious or sarcastic. In order to be effective, it must be stated with the utmost sincerity, which can come only from believing that it is the systemic truth of the family. We have found that no matter how absurd a message may sound, someone in the family usually confirms its validity, as in the case of the Allen father, who confirms that it is better for his wife to fight with her son than with him. This has led us to the comforting conclusion that it is difficult, if not impossible, to surpass the absurdity of an emotional system.

The Miller family was referred for treatment after the mother had made a suicide attempt and then refused in the hospital to give up her pills. The event that precipitated the mother's suicide attempt was a scuffle over the couple's "problem son," Gary, 11. The mother had been trying unsuccessfully to discipline him. She called to the father for help, but he was asleep and did not come, whereupon she went to the bathroom and took an overdose of sleeping pills.

During the past two years the father has suffered a series of heart attacks that left him with an "inoperable" heart condition. His doctor ordered him to stop working, and he now stays at home, a semi-invalid. The family is beset with every kind of problem—financial, legal, physical, social, and emotional—and live from crisis to crisis.

Not only is Gary's problem an old problem, but the conflict between the parents is of many years' duration. Five years previously they were in marital therapy and, according to them, were told their marriage was hopeless and they should seek a divorce. Instead, they placed Gary in individual therapy for three years. The parents are involved in a power struggle around every issue of their lives: where they should live, such as in an apartment or a house, near to his parents or to hers; how much money they should spend; who should do what around the house; where they should spend their vacation; and who should discipline the children. All arguments are settled by default. The person who *can* do it, *does* do it. The family rule is, "Never say *won't;* say *can't.*"

For many years Gary has been at the center of this power struggle. The cycle that maintains the symptom is as follows: Gary will misbehave in some small way, and the mother will become angry at the father for not disciplining him. Rather than express her anger, she will attempt to discipline Gary in such a way as to escalate his misbehavior. She will then become sick in the process, and the father will be forced to take over. The father will then have an angina attack from the exertion, and both parents will end up blaming Gary. Physical symptoms are used as a means of control, and each parent keeps escalating. The father is now ahead in the contest because of the seriousness of his heart condition. The ante being raised, the mother retaliates by increasing the severity of her colitis, back pains, and depression, culminating in a suicide attempt.

The contest between the parents might best be described as "he who loses, wins," the winner not having to take responsibility for running the family. It is literally a fight to the death, with the mother desperately trying to produce a symptom more serious than her husband's heart condition. In the middle of attempting to discipline Gary, she will suddenly fall to the floor with an attack of colitis and, according to her, "lie there bleeding for hours, unable to get up." Or she will develop pains in her back and have to go to bed for a week in traction. After each of the father's hospitalizations she hospitalizes herself with one of her symptoms. Periodically she will threaten to have Gary placed, screaming, "If he stays here, either I'll kill him or he'll kill me," and the cycle continues without end.

The children duplicate the contest between the parents, with the younger sister, Sally, nine, developing physical symptoms like her mother to control her brother and parents. She has a repertoire of dramatic ailments, such as nightmares, insomnia, fainting spells, stomach pains, headaches, and will declare tearfully in a session, "What about me? I have terrible problems, you know; I'm emotionally disturbed too," which will prompt the mother to ask if she should not be in individual therapy.

Direct interventions, such as trying to get the parents to work cooperatively in establishing consistent controls for Gary or communicating their own needs directly rather than indirectly, are doomed to failure. There is always a different reason why they are unable to follow through on suggestions, or, if they do, why the suggestions are not helpful. The contest is gaining its power from being played "outside awareness" on the part of the participants and therefore does not respond to suggestions, explanations, or confrontations.

When the decision is made to use a systemic paradox, the therapist is faced with the difficult task of redefining the deadly contest positively. This is done by describing the power maneuvers as being motivated by love and caring. The therapist reads a message from the group stating that in this family people show their love for one another by being miserable so that other family members can feel more fortunate than they.

This message is dramatized within the family sessions at every opportunity, both in the parental system and in the sibling subsystem. For example, during one session Sally talks about having won the lead in the school play. Although she wanted it desperately, she complains about getting it, as now the other children are jealous of her. She thus manages to turn a winning experience into a losing one. After a consultation with the group, the therapist returns with the following message: "Sally is wise to complain and cry at the moment of her greatest triumph, which is winning the lead in the school play. By not appearing joyous, she is following her mother's example of not allowing herself to feel pleasure. This is for fear of making other family members feel less fortunate. We believe, therefore, that it is only fitting that Father and Gary encourage Sally and Mother to be unhappy, because in this way they will show their appreciation for what Sally and Mother are doing for family closeness."

The family's reaction can best be described as one of incredulity. For the first time the mother mentions the word *change*. "Isn't there some way to change that? It sounds very bad ... Isn't there some way we could all feel good, not bad?" The therapist questions the wisdom of this, since feeling bad is their way of showing their love for one another.

At the beginning of the following session, the therapist asks if they have followed through on the recommendation.

Sally: Oh, yes, now I remember. We should not allow ourselves to feel happy because the others might feel bad.

Gary: It says in my mother's psychology book that if one person is unhappy and the other is happy, it'll make him feel worse, so the other should become sad to make him not feel as bad.

Papp: The group feels that's what goes on in this family and that you show your love for each other by being unhappy and miserable and sick.

Mother: Isn't there some way to change it somehow or—break the pattern?

Papp: Why would you want to do that?

Mother: Because it seems like a sick way of doing things.

Papp (to father): What do you think?

Father: I don't know—I don't quite understand—uh—I don't quite see the whole thing.

Papp: Mm. Gary?

Gary: In my mother's psychology book it says there should be shifts. I mean we should switch over—I mean one person should feel bad to make another feel better (*looking embarrassed by the idea*), but I don't agree with it.

Papp (deciding to prescribe the contest more explicitly): I would like to suggest something. This may sound crazy, but I'd like to suggest it anyway. The next time Gary throws a temper tantrum, Sally, what I'd like you to do is—to feel bad. (*Everyone laughs.*) Just see if it works. Do you know the first sign?

Sally: I can hear his screams. He moans and groans and whines.

Papp: At that moment when you see he is going to have one of his weekly temper tantrums, could you act worse—start to cry, start to complain about friends in school, um? (*Sally giggles.*)

Gary: I'd know she was doing that.

Papp: It doesn't matter. Would you do that for him?

Sally: Yes, but once in a while you be nice to me.

Papp: We'll talk about how he can repay you later, but first let's see whether this will be helpful to him, okay? When he first shows signs that he's about to have a tantrum, you create a rumpus. I think that will be helpful to him.

Gary: And vice versa.

Papp: Are you willing to do it?

Sally: I'll try, but I want him to pay me back.

Gary: I know how. Her language is foul and Dad doesn't like it, and she is sent upstairs—

Papp: You mean, when she's in trouble, you'll rescue her by acting up?

Gary: Yeah, is that what you mean?

Sally: That's paying me back.

Gary: That's what I meant it for.

Papp: That's very nice of you.

Gary: I didn't mean it to be nice, but—

Papp: You didn't?

Gary: No. (*Parents laugh.*) I object to this whole thing.

Papp: What would you do if she begins to throw a fit?

Gary: I would begin to cry and complain—but—but, as I said, I'm against this whole thing.

Sally: What happens if one person disregards this request?

Gary: Yeah. Like if one person doesn't do his share of the work.

Papp: Then suppose the other person reminded him. If you start to throw a temper tantrum, you could say to Sally, "Please rescue me." (*Much laughter.*)

Gary: What if I help her one day and she doesn't help me—I mean, should I remind her?

Papp: Yes, remind her, and you remind him.

Sally then offers to sacrifice herself by not showing her brother how good she feels about being in the school play.

Sally: I can keep him happy by forgetting what's happening in school. The play will only last a few days. Everyone feels good when they have a secret of some kind, or something that—uh, hum—in a way they're helping someone else. They feel better, they feel good. But I would show whatever's bad on the outside and keep my good on the inside.

Papp: I see, just to help Gary. Don't you think that's nice of her?

Gary (noncommittally): Mm.

Sally: If you don't think it's nice, I just won't do it.

Gary: It won't work because you've already told me you're going to pretend to feel bad.

Sally: But you don't know when. Don't worry. I won't let you feel bad. I'll keep you happy.

Gary: But you can't if I know you will.

Sally: You'll forget all about it, don't worry.

Gary: I doubt it.

Sally: Try hard not to keep it in mind. Don't worry. On the outside I'll feel bad, but on the inside I'll feel good. How can you know how I feel on the inside? You can't.

By being openly prescribed, the secret contest is robbed of its lethal power and takes on the quality of an innocent game. Having been defined as being motivated by caring and protectiveness, it is now being played in that spirit. The therapist then turns to the parents and prescribes their contest.

Papp: When one of you is feeling down, how can the other one go down further to allow the one to come up?

Father: I don't know.

Papp: What are the signs?

Father: I tire more easily.

Papp (to mother): Can you make him feel better about his physical condition by your tiring sooner than he does and by—

Father: She does.

Papp: She does?

Father: Yes. She always tires before me.

Papp: Then what about feeling worse physically than he does to make him feel strong and healthy. Can you do that?

Mother: I don't think that works.

Father: She does.

Papp: She does?

Father: She does to an extent. Between her back and her colitis.

Papp: Maybe.

Father: We plan to do things and when the day comes she doesn't feel like it, and we cancel our plans so it's another boring day.

Papp: How do you convey to your husband that you're in a worse state than he is?

Mother: I don't know . . . if I am, I am. Why shouldn't everyone feel good at once?

Both parents and children then collude to dismiss the contest. They talk about all feeling good and doing things together. This ends up with the father relating a recent anecdote about buying tickets for a play, but having an argument about which play, and the mother getting sick so they couldn't go.

Papp: I don't think both feeling good together is the answer.

The children try again to work out a compromise solution for their parents, which goes nowhere.

Papp (to children): You're trying to work it out so they're both happy, but I don't think that will work. (*To husband.*) You must get more unhappy when you see her down in order to bring her up. And you have to get more unhappy to bring your husband up.

Father: You're saying if one feels unhappy, the other person will forget how unhappy he feels, to help the other person?

Papp: That's right, that's right.

Father: I've seen these shifts. I've seen things like that. Not so much now as when I was sicker. When I felt bad a number of times, you have felt very bad. One of us had to do something—prepare a meal or something like that—and I was already bad and you all of a sudden say you're worse, so I would have to go make the dinner. And I would be angry at you because you always seem to find yourself sick when I'm sick. That is what I think we're getting at.

Papp: But look, it was helpful to you because you got up and did it.

Father: Just because I did it doesn't mean I felt any better.

Papp (to mother): Some place, deep down inside, you were being helpful to your husband.

Father: Because it got me up?

Papp (to mother): Deep down inside you knew if you felt worse than he did, it would help him, and you're very protective of him. And when do you protect her like that?

Father: You're saying when do I do it consciously?

Papp: Well, or unconsciously.

Father: I may be doing it subconsciously.

Papp: Okay. It doesn't matter. See if you can figure out when you do it unconsciously. When do you feel worse in order to make her feel better when she's down?

Father: When I feel worse, I don't think I put it on.

Papp: You're not as protective of her as she is of you?

Father: When she feels bad, I try to take over some of the burden.

The father then describes taking over the disciplining of Gary.

Papp: In a sense you don't have to try as hard as your wife does because of your health. You're always worse off than she.

Father: I don't think recently I've felt in poorer condition than she.

The therapist excuses herself for a consultation and returns with a message of reinforcement from the group.

Papp: "The group would like to applaud mother for her efforts to be more unhappy than her husband. Because of her great love for him, she knows that the best way to energize him when he feels low is to be even more dispirited than he so that he can rise to the occasion by helping her. She knows if she were to become energetic and take over, father might become more of an invalid.

"Therefore, we recommend that the moment she sees that her husband is tempted to give in to his illness, she let herself become more miserable than he. In case she misses the signal, he should let her know in whatever way he feels is appropriate.

"We also recommend that Sally and Gary continue to provide their parents with a good example by rescuing each other when either is in trouble."

The hidden power struggle is no longer hidden. It is rendered impotent through its exposure and scheduling. The denial and subterfuge surrounding it are replaced with conscious intention, which makes it difficult to continue it in the same virulent way.

17 Strengths

A therapist is working with the Baos, a Vietnamese family composed of a widowed mother in her late thirties and four preadolescent children, who have been in the United States for four years. The hierarchy of the family has been distorted because, as often happens, the Bao children have become more skilled than their mother in using English and negotiating the everyday events of the new culture. The therapist, Jay Lappin, has trouble finding strengths in the mother to highlight because her difficulty with English restricts their communication. In a flash of inspiration and despair, he teaches the family to play "Simon Says." But they are to play it in Vietnamese, with the mother in charge.

In the ensuing month this game, and variations on it, become the field in which the mother teaches both the children and the therapist about Vietnamese culture, geography, and cooking. At the same time, since she has to translate for the therapist, her understanding of English and of American culture improves. The children begin to remember Vietnamese and use the recovered language proudly, while Mrs. Bao begins to use her new expertise to coach recently arrived immigrants in managing the American welfare bureaucracy. This family teaches the therapist something fundamental about therapy: every family has elements in their own culture which, if understood and utilized, can become levers to actualize and expand the family members' behavioral repertory.

Unfortunately, we therapists have not assimilated this axiom. Though we pay lip service to the strengths of the family, and talk about it as the matrix of development and healing, we are trained as psychological sleuths. Our instincts are to "search and destroy": pinpoint the psychological disorder, label it, and eradicate it. We are the "experts." We are the specialized personnel who have earned our credentials to defend the normal by developing and maintaining a typology that frames deviancy as mental illness. Ironically, this job of policing deviance is organized in relation to a model of the normal that is vague and undifferentiated at best. Like the sorcerer's apprentice, we use a mixture of wisdom, technology, and ignorance. Imprisoned in the prevalent cultural mores of our institutional contexts, we explore pathology like a physician trying to identify a virus, defining and redefining deviance. Every few years the mental health movement goes through a ritual of revising its diagnostic categories. Some illnesses are expurgated, and those behaviors are returned to the category of the normal. The most recent such ritual returned to health all the homosexuals who, the day before, had been relegated to the closets of the mentally ill.

FAMILY DEFICITS

Fortunately for family therapy, therapists have not been able to develop diagnostic categories for families that can pigeonhole some family forms as normal and others as deviant; with any luck, we never will develop them. Yet we have been handicapped by the pervasive view that polarizes "the family" and "the individual," framing life as a heroic struggle between the part and the whole. Family therapists know that the human being is a holon, but somehow, the belonging that is necessary to that holon is framed as a defeat: a loss of self.

At its extreme, this cultural and esthetic preference for the individual-as-a-whole treats the family as the enemy of the individual. Ashley Montagu regards the family as "an institution for the systematic production of physical and mental illness in the members." Susan Sontag views the modern nuclear family as "a psychological and moral disaster . . . a prison of sexual repression, a playing field of inconsistent moral laxity, a museum of possessiveness, a guilt-producing factory, a school of selfishness."[1]

The modern person, living in a society that is less and less predictable, bracing himself for a world that is forever more complex, expresses his struggle with society in his relationship within his own family, which is a microcosm of society at large. The poet Philip Larkin concludes:

They fuck you up, your mum and dad,
　They may not mean to, but they do.
They fill you with the faults they had
　And add some extra, just for you.

But they were fucked up in their turn
　By fools in old-style hats and coats
Who half the time were soppy-stern
　And half at one another's throats.

Man hands on misery to man,
　It deepens like the coastal shelf.
Get out as quickly as you can
　And don't have any kids yourself.[2]

The psychiatrist R. D. Laing, who has pursued a crusade against the family in defense of the individual, observes, "The initial act of brutality against the average child is mother's first kiss." In describing his own family, Laing remarks: "From as far back as I can remember, I tried to figure out what was going on between these people. If I believed one, I couldn't believe anyone else." Of his father, he notes: "My father regarded his father as having murdered his mother 'systematically' over the years. The last time he 'ever set foot in the door of our house' (according to my parents), the radio was on; he sat down and told my mother to turn it off. My father told my mother to do nothing of the kind. Old Pa, as my father's father was called, told my mother to turn it off. And so on. Eventually my father said, 'This is my house, and the radio will stay on unless I say so!' Old Pa said, 'Don't speak to your father like that!' My father said, 'Get up and get out!' Old Pa reminded him once more whom he was speaking to. My father pointed out he knew very well whom he was speaking to, that was why he was telling him to get up and get out. Old Pa made no move, whereupon my father went to throw him out 'by the scruff of the neck.' The fight was on. Old Pa in his fifties, my father in his thirties. The fight went on all over the house. Eventually my father pinned Old Pa on his back across the bed, and smashed him across the face until blood was flowing. He then dragged him to the bathroom, rolled him into the bath, turned the cold water on him, heaved him out drenched with blood and water, dragged him to the door, kicked him out and threw his cap after him. Then he stood at the window and waited to see how he would manage to stagger or crawl away. 'He held himself up very well,' Dad said. 'You've got to hand it to him.' "[3] But what Laing provides here is a construction that supports his world view. He presents certain narrow aspects of the family experience as all-encompassing universals. Clearly other components in the transactions of family members could have been selected instead.

The family therapist Andrew Ferber describes his family in an equally narrow fashion: "Betty, my sister, is five years my junior. Although an attractive and intelligent child, she was the family scapegoat. She was neglected and rejected. I was originally her torturer, then her hero and protector. My father would form an alliance with me against my mother, who was represented as dull and stupid. My mother formed an alliance with me against my father, who was called self-indulgent and neglectful. I served as a bridge between my mother and father and my sister. I was raised as a star and a show-off and reveled in it. I was a charming monster. We were all too self-centered, isolated from each other and from both extended families.[4]

These two constructions, based on selective memories, represent two psychiatrists' induction into the mores of the culture that they inhabit: a culture that tends to focus on deficits and deviancy, and which yearns for the knight on the white horse who will rid society of its dragons. The immensely complex nature of the human niche in space and time is reduced to the Homeric simplicity of the epic struggle of "man the hero."

FAMILY CONTRIBUTIONS

Family therapists are now modifying their perspective and looking for the contributions of the family, for it is the relatively unsung characteristics of families—the nurturing, the caring, the supportive transactions—that ensure survival in a complex world. This is so much a part of reality that it is simply taken for granted.

Stand in a matinée line for *The Empire Strikes Back,* full of families of all sizes, shapes, and colors and watch the small transactions. Watch the eight-year-old black girl with a complicated hair-do and a brilliant smile coach her three-year-old sister, who is singing the alphabet while her father and grandmother nod approval. Watch the "dumb blond" mother who, while waiting with her three boys, aged six to nine, and her seven-year-old niece, who lives with her and is "like my own," is combing the children's hair in four strikingly different styles. Notice the Jewish grandfather and his eight-year-old grandson just standing there, equally eager to see the show. After the movie, listen to the parents trying to explain the ending to their children. How is it possible for the hero, young Luke Skywalker, to be the son of the malevolent Darth Vader, and still be a good guy?

Family life is not the stuff of epics. But in its small transactions, which escape the synthesizing power of a Laing or a Sontag, the family shows what it can accomplish.

Consider the Gage family in Worcester, as described by Jane Howard: "Nick Gage—his sisters and kinfolk usually refer to him by his full name—came from Greece at the age of nine with high resolve. Talented in mathematics, he thought he would become an engineer. When he won an essay contest, he changed his mind and decided on a writing career instead. He started to earn money. He also helped his immigrating relatives. Streaming across the Atlantic in growing numbers, they needed someone to figure out tax returns, citizenship papers, driver's licenses, and other American obstacles. Someone had to interpret their new country to them. The someone was Nick.

"So it still goes. 'Nobody would ever think of buying property without consulting Nick first,' one cousin said. He arranges immigration papers, advises about all manner of things, and works so hard on his own projects that Papou is afraid he will squeeze his brains . . .

"His sister Lilia, who helps her husband with the pizza, doesn't look much like Nick except for her eyes and her hair, which, like his, is light brown . . . She is as central to her clan as her brother and their father. She provides a service no clan can do without: she is its switchboard. She is the one who knows, at any given time, where her eighty closest relatives are and what, more or less, is on their minds. She knows who is about to have surgery, who might be on the brink of engagement or marriage or divorce, who may be having what she calls "the trouble with the school," and who has reservations to fly to, or return from, Athens. Someone in this clan is always packing or unpacking a suitcase load of presents: sheets and pillowcases and towels and shawls for the other side of the Atlantic; jars of holy water and charms to pin on children's clothing to ward off the evil eye for this side."[5]

A different, but somehow similar, view of families comes from John Elderkin Bell's description of a small hospital in Cameroon: "In this four-bed room . . . the beds are narrow, but there is room on one of them for an old man patient and his wife to sit together most of the day. Occasionally she leaves to prepare some food in one of the kitchens at the back of the hospital. Today, she was given some stew by an old man in a bed on the other side of the room. He signaled to her that he had too much—he didn't speak—and she took a bowl and brought some of his stew back for herself and her husband. They sat together and silently ate it from the same bowl with two spoons. Probably they were silent because the stew had come originally from the woman now sitting on the floor by the next bed eating her own. She was the mother of the college boy lying on that bed.

"This mother had made a room for herself under her student son's bed. She had spread a mat for sleeping, stored her teakettle, a lantern, a primus stove, a teapot, and a pan under the head of the bed. Over the bottom rung of the bedstead she had hung her sweater. She had just poured stew for her son, who was resting against an embroidered pillow she had brought from home. Behind his head was a more elaborately patterned pillow, also from home, and above that a hospital cupboard where were stored their dishes of their food.

"Near this room is a four-bed room for children. Each child has his mother with him. Some are very sick. Most of the mothers sleep in the beds with the children, to protect them, to keep them warm, to watch over them, and to continue the pattern of home where the mother sleeps with the young children."

In the next room is a government employee. "On the bed beside him sat his pregnant wife who had been with him all the time since he came in a week ago. They had a crib moved in for their infant son, and the father's sister had come along to help look after the baby . . . this man had probably sought a government position after getting his high school education, not only for the salary, which is low, but for the possible power to control appointments in order to take care of his relatives and to serve the public in some role where a fee may be charged. The tradition of looking after one's own is so strong that making provision for the extended family through one's position is regarded as ethical and as a fulfilling of moral duty. There is so little public pressure against such practices that there is fierce competition to secure a government appointment and to maintain such an advantageous position."[6]

The small transactions that occur in these wards—the preparing of food, the sitting silently together, the giving up of ordinary routines to care for a relative in need—all these are familiar elements of family life that exist anywhere. Nick Gage's family in Worcester is, in this respect, very similar to the Minuchin family in Argentina, in Israel, and in the United States, to Bell's families in Cameroon and to the family to which Betty MacDonald returned after leaving a miserable marriage in the worst of the Great Depression: "It's a wonderful thing to know that you can come home anytime from anywhere and just open the door and belong. That everybody will shift until you fit and that from that day on it's a matter of sharing everything. When you share your money, your clothes and your food with a mother, a brother and three sisters, your portion may be meagre but by the same token when you share unhappiness, loneliness and anxiety about the future with a mother, a brother and three sisters, there isn't much left for you."[7]

In every family there are positives. Positives are transmitted from the family of origin to the new family, and from there to the next generation. Despite mistakes, unhappiness, and pain, there are also pleasures: spouses and children give to each other in ways that are growth-encouraging and supportive, contributing to each other's sense of competence and worth. Every family is like Laing's and Ferber's in some ways, but it is also like Nick Gage's. To paraphrase Aesop's fable, the family is the best and the worst that humans have.

The orientation of family therapists toward "constructing a reality" that highlights deficits is therefore being challenged. Family therapists are finding that an exploration of strengths is essential to challenge family dysfunctions. The work of Virginia Satir, with its emphasis on growth, is oriented toward a search for normal alternatives. So is the work of Ivan Nagy, with its emphasis on positive connotations and his exploration of the family value system. Carl Whitaker's technique of challenging the positions of family members and introducing role diffusion springs from his belief that out of this therapeutically induced chaos the family members can discover latent strength. Jay Haley and Chloe Madanes' view that the symptom is organized to protect the family and Mara Selvini-Palazzoli's paradoxical interventions all point toward family strengths.

Physicians working with cancer victims and other seriously ill patients are looking at the family as a reservoir for healing and strength. Harold Wise assembles family members and friends for sessions called therapeutic family reunions, lasting from a day to a week. Ross and Joan Speck, collaborating with Wise, apply network therapy to families where there is a cancer or heart disease diathesis. Work on long-standing family grievances, mourning, or feuds, they are convinced, can tighten the bonds between people and produce a helping and healing effect throughout the system, prolonging the life of the index patient.

In Milton Erickson's work with individuals, he addressed himself consistently to the "fact" that individuals have a reservoir of wisdom, learned and forgotten but still available. He suggested that his patients explore alternative ways of organizing their experience without exploring the etiology or dynamics of the dysfunction. This search for valid and functional alternatives of transaction is also applicable in family therapy, for the family is an organism that has available a larger repertory of ways of organizing experience than those it ordinarily uses. One strategy is therefore to bypass an exploration of the historical underpinnings of dysfunctional transactions and to take a shortcut of exploring other, more complex modes of transacting that promise healthier functioning.

Families come to a family therapist when they are stuck in a situation which requires changes that the family does not see as available in its repertory. At this point, the family focuses on the stress of one of its members and narrows its exploration for alternatives by defining that member as deviant. In the period preceding their arrival at the therapist's office, all of the family members have been searching for the cause of the illness. In effect, their shared worldview has narrowed and crystallized to a concentration on pathology. A challenge to that view which focuses on the healing capacities of the family may result in a transformation of the reality that the family apprehends. The challenge can be related either to the family's response to the identified patient or to the family's use of alternatives.

RESPONSE TO IDENTIFIED PATIENT

Cases of handicapped children are especially revealing, since in families with children with chronic conditions there is a tendency on the part of the family to organize themselves around the child's weaknesses, minimizing her competence. The Thomas family is a case in point. Thirty minutes into a session, the therapist helps Pauline, an 11-year-old asthmatic who is the identified patient, describe the way in which the family members, in their attempt to protect her, increase her sense of panic when an attack starts. The therapist's emphasis here is on Pauline's ability to describe the interpersonal transactions and on her skill at reading faces and understanding people.

Minuchin: You know something, Pauline, in this family everybody watches you. Everybody is very worried about you. Are you also worried about yourself? Are you scared?
Pauline: Sort of.
Minuchin: At which point of the asthma attack do you get scared?
Pauline: When the attack starts.
Minuchin: I like that. You answered the question. So immediately when you start to breathe heavy, you get scared? And what do you do then?
Pauline: I drink juices.

Minuchin: And then?

Pauline: Sit under the air conditioner.

Minuchin: And then? What do you do then?

Pauline: Sometimes I lie down.

Minuchin: What happens when you lie down? Does Mom or Uncle Jim or Grandma come to talk to you?

Pauline: My Uncle Jim.

Minuchin: And is your Uncle Jim worried?

Pauline: Yes.

Minuchin: How do you know he's worried? Look at him. Is he worried now?

Pauline: I can't tell with the glasses on. (*Uncle takes off his glasses.*) No.

Minuchin: But you know when his face is worried. How does his face look when he is worried?

Pauline: Like mad.

Minuchin: Do you notice that in his eyes, or in his mouth, or in his forehead?

Pauline: He gets red in the face.

Minuchin: And when Mommy comes, is she worried?

Pauline: Yes.

Minuchin: How do you know that she's worried? Look at Mommy's face. Is she worried now?

Pauline: No.

Minuchin: How does she look when she's worried?

Pauline: Sad.

Minuchin: Sad. And do you notice that in her eyes or in her mouth? Where do you notice that she's sad?

Pauline: Her eyes.

Minuchin: Her eyes. She kind of looks sad in her eyes. Sometimes Grandma comes if you have an attack? How does she look?

Pauline: Mad.

Minuchin: And where do you see that? In her eyes, or in where?

Pauline: Her face.

Minuchin: How do you see that she's mad?

Pauline: She's fussing.

Minuchin: Do you think she's mad, or do you think she's worried?

Pauline: Worried.

Minuchin: She's worried. And she fusses when she worries. How does she fuss? What does she do?

Pauline: It's, "Why don't you call and let me know she's in the hospital?"

Minuchin: To whom does she say that? To Mother?

Pauline: Yeah.

Minuchin: What about Aunt Sarah? How do you know if she is worried or not?

Pauline: Because she kept asking me if I was feeling all right, and I said yes. But I wasn't feeling all right.

Minuchin: You mean she's kind of watching you and she's concerned. So everybody is watching you pretty close, huh? Do you like it that everybody's watching you so close?

Pauline: Yeah.

Minuchin: You do like it. So that then you are safe because everybody's watching you.

Pauline: Yes.

In this painstakingly slow segment, the therapist puts the girl into contact with each one of the family members, describing the way in which she experiences their moods and affects in relationship to herself. This is probably a unique experience for a family that has responded to the identified patient only in terms of her needs and her fears. The therapist's emphasis on the patient's competence changes the way in which she experiences her relationship to the rest of the family. As a result, by the end of this exchange some of her statements become more elaborated ("Because she kept asking me if I was feeling all right, and I said yes. But I wasn't feeling all right"). They are much longer and more descriptive than the ones that the girl usually produces in the session. The rest of the family is kept passive, as listeners, while the girl is made the central person, communicating about each one of them. This is a change in the nature of their usual transactions, one that emphasizes competence and strength instead of pathology and the need for protection.

Minuchin: What do you feel before the attack begins? Sometimes children with asthma feel a tightness in the chest. Sometimes they feel a slight headache. Sometimes they feel breathless, uncomfortable. But you're not accustomed to listening to your body. You wait for your mom or your grandma, or your uncles, to feel worried for you. I want you to learn to listen to your body. What I am saying is very difficult, and I don't know that I am coming across. Do you know what I am saying?

Pauline: No.

Minuchin (putting his hands on Pauline's chest and holding tight): What did you feel?

Pauline: I feel tension.

Minuchin: Okay. You felt your body. Don't breathe. (*Pinches Pauline's nostrils, closing them.*) What did you feel?

Pauline: I could not breathe.

Minuchin: You felt something within you. You felt like you wanted to breathe and couldn't?

Pauline: Yeah.

Minuchin (again closing Pauline's nostrils): So you felt your body, okay? Sometimes before you have an attack, you will feel something like that. What will you do if I don't stop closing your nose? (*Pauline opens her mouth and breathes.*) Of course. You said, "This crazy man is closing my nose. I will breathe." Didn't you do that? So you changed, you did something.

The girl begins to inhale and exhale deeply. The therapist and patient engage in five minutes of exercises, in which Pauline is asked to pay attention to her proprioceptive responses.

Minuchin: Do you do your exercises with your mom or do you do them alone?

Pauline: Sometimes with my mom and sometimes by myself.

Minuchin: Why do you do it with your mom?

Pauline: So she can tell if they're working or not.

Minuchin: You can't tell? (*To the family.*) We are having again and again the same thing. That she is relying on other people to help her. (*To Pauline.*) You are loving and you have a lovely mind and you think very nicely and I like the way in which you told me how everybody else in the family helps you, how they are worried. But you need to help your family not to talk for you and not to be scared for you. Tell it back to me so I will know that you understand. What did I say?

Pauline: I have to do all those things by myself. Talk more.

Minuchin: I want you to tell that to your mommy now.

Pauline: Mommy, I know how to think by myself.

Mother: Well, I want you to show me then. Let's see as of today.

Minuchin: Talk to your grandma also so she will know.

Pauline: Grandma, I know how to think by myself.

Grandmother: Okay. (*Pauline goes and gets close to each member of the family and repeats a variation on the same theme: "I don't need your help to talk for myself."*)

At the end of the session, the therapist engages the girl in a series of exercises and activities related to increasing her ability to perceive proprioceptive feedback. This transaction emphasizes the girl's functioning alone, listening to her own body and becoming increasingly more involved with herself, instead of listening to all the family members who observe her. In the end, the therapist offers a ritual to reinforce the message, and the session finishes with the identified patient engaged in a ritualistic transaction with each family member in which she declares her ability, her right, and her obligation to function independently. A follow-up three months after this session establishes that there was no attack of asthma during this period.

Bill Simon is a 13-year-old blind boy who was referred to the clinic because he is destructive; he destroys radios and other household instruments. His parents, who cannot control him, are concerned that he may hurt his three-month-old infant brother. Minuchin, who is a consultant in the case, is impressed by the fact that both the therapist, H. Goa, and the father use a language full of nonverbal modifers and sprinkled with words that imply *seeing,* apparently unaware that Bill's way of apprehending the world is necessarily different from theirs. Minuchin sits close to Bill so that the boy can experience his proximity and can touch him. The mother is not present in this session, as she needs to remain at home with the infant.

Minuchin: You are an expert in something in which I am not an expert, Bill. You are an expert in understanding things without seeing. You see, I see, so I don't know many things. How do you understand objects?

Bill: Because I can touch them. You don't have to see objects to understand.

Minuchin: I don't know. You can touch them, and what happens when you touch them? For instance, what is that? (*Hands Bill a book.*)

Bill: I know what that is. It's a book.

Minuchin: Can you tell me more about that? I just want to know how a person that doesn't see understands things.

Bill: Well, I don't know what the book is called, because I can't read and it's print.

Minuchin: What else? Tell me what else you know about this book. Is it a large book?

Bill: It's a small book, pretty small.

Minuchin: Yeah. And it's a hard cover?

Bill: No, it isn't. It's a soft cover.

Minuchin: What else can you tell me about this book?

Bill: It has many pages. I don't know how many it has.

Minuchin: Okay. So that is how you understand that object: you touch it. Do you smell it also?

Bill: No.

Minuchin: Can you make it make a sound? I just want to know if you can hear a book or not. (*Rustles the pages of the book.*)

Bill: Yes, I can hear the book.

Minuchin: You can hear the book. Okay. So how can you understand a child? How can you understand your brother without seeing him?

Bill: I can hear him cry, but I don't understand what kind of voice he's going to have or anything.

Minuchin: Does he cry differently at different times? Does he have a soft cry and a hard cry?

Bill: He starts to get mad and he starts to cry up and up further until we know that something must be wrong with him, or he's hungry, or he's wet.

Minuchin: Of course.

The consultant expresses his ignorance of the identified patient's world but his willingness to learn, presenting to both father and son a model of the relationship between a handicapped child and an adult that challenges the family program, since it assumes competence in the blind child.

Minuchin: I want you to hear what I have to say to Dr. Goa. When I was listening to you, Bill, I began to think that really I don't understand how you understand things, because I watch to understand many things. And you probably have other ways. And I would like to know if you can help your father and work out with your father some way in which your father will help you to understand your brother. How large are the baby's hands?

Bill: They're small. They're not real large.

Minuchin: How do you know that?

Bill: 'Cause I touched him.

Minuchin: Did you touch him all over the body? Do you understand how the body is formed?

Bill: I don't understand how the inside is formed, but the outside I've touched.

Minuchin (to father): I think that Bill can teach you and Dr. Goa and me certain things we cannot understand. And I'm wondering, Bill, if you are stingy because you don't teach your father some of the ways in which you understand the world that your father cannot understand.

Again the consultant challenges the notion of the child's incompetence, framing the father-son transaction in terms of the son's withholding instead of the child's deficiency.

Minuchin: Am I close to you or am I distant from you?

Bill: You're close because I can hear you.

Minuchin: You can hear me. How do you understand me?

Bill: Your voice. Your accent, really.

Minuchin: Yeah. What accent do I have?

Bill: I don't know. Sort of a Phillipine. Sounds like it.

Minuchin: Is it similar to the accent of Dr. Goa?

Minuchin: No. It isn't.

Minuchin: It isn't. What accent has Dr. Goa?

Bill: I guess it's Spanish. I don't know what you call it.

Minuchin: Spanish is absolutely correct. My accent is also Spanish.

Bill: Then I'm not right.

Minuchin: You're also right. The Filipino has a lot of Spanish. Am I young, or am I old?

Bill: I can't tell if you're young or old.

Minuchin: How could you?

Bill: By your voice? If you're old, you have a real old voice, but if you're young, you have a real young voice.

Minuchin: And my voice, how old is my voice?

Bill: Sounds like forty.

Minuchin: That's very good. How old is your father's?

Bill: Sounds like thirty-three.

Minuchin: How old are you?

Father: Thirty-four.

Minuchin: So my voice is older than your father's. You see, you know a lot of things.

Bill: I don't know about the baby's voice until it gets bigger.

Father: That's interesting, the way he thinks.

Minuchin: I think, Bill, that you are stingy. I think that you have a knowledge of hearing and a knowledge of touch that your father doesn't have because he sees. You taught him how you understand me; you have better hearing than he does.

The consultant and the therapist agree that Bill should teach his father how to go around the room blindfolded, since Bill has a sense of space that the father does not share.

Goa: Your dad is going to close his eyes.

Bill: I'm already blind. Don't blindfold me.

Goa: You don't need to be nervous about that. Your daddy is going to close his eyes, and you're going to lead him around the room and discover what's in the room. Okay? So he's going to close his eyes. He's not going to see anymore. Okay? Remember that your dad doesn't see. You have to protect him.

Bill (taking his father's hand and moving around the room, guiding his father): There's a chair over here.

Goa: Show him. Don't forget about your dad.

Bill: This is the door. This is another chair over here. And this is the door.

Goa: Don't go out of the room. Just show him what is in here.

Bill: And there's some chairs. I bet there's a closet over here.

The session ends with the father and son sharing a new reality, the discovery of a relationship in which the son's competence is acknowledged and the father can accept learning from his handicapped son. This change can realign the positions of all family members by giving Bill more participation in family activities and demanding more responsible behavior from him.

A similar strategy has been used by Sam Scott in his work with deaf children. These children, who are taught to sign in a school for hearing-impaired children, find at home an environment in which the rest of the family speak and hear but do not know how to sign. The educational program organizes the children to have contact with other children and teachers at school but reduces their ability to communicate at home.

Scott therefore assigns each child as a teacher of her siblings and parents in "classes" at which the family learns how to sign in order to communicate with the child. This complete reversal of the position of the handicapped child in her family has a profound significance for the way in which the family functions. The same orientation toward exploring positives among family members underlies all the other techniques.

TRANSACTING ALTERNATIVES

Families involved in unresolved conflicts tend to become stereotyped in the repetitive mishandling of interpersonal transactions, with the result that the family members narrow their observation of each other and focus on the deficits in the family. When they come to treatment, they present the more dysfunctional aspects of themselves; these are the areas seen as relevant to therapy. Family members also tend to reserve their more competent ways of functioning for extrafamilial holons. Their utilization of self in the dysfunctional family organism becomes narrower and less complex. The family therapist should not respond to the family as if their presentation of the dysfunctional stereotypes were the whole of the family. The dysfunctional components are merely those segments of the full family potential that are, at this point, most available to the family organism.

If the family therapist is an enthusiastic psychopathologist, he will respond to the morsels of pathology that the family presents and be misled into observing only the less competent parts of the family organism. If he expands his focus of exploration, however, he will find that the family has alternatives that can be mobilized. The Horowitz couple, for instance, presents their symmetrical competitiveness and their lack of mutuality. The therapist, watching their dysfunctional transactions, says to them, "Okay, I have seen that you are experts at disqualifying each other. Can you now get out of this particular corner?" There is in the therapist's message an acknowledgment of the present transactions but also an implication of the availability of unused alternatives that moves the couple to explore them. The therapist's statement is based on his belief that the family as an organism has the potential for more complex functioning than that they are presenting at the moment. There is no exploration of the dysfunctional components; instead, there is an invitation to explore alternatives.

The therapist may observe during a session that the behavior of the family members is within the range of the normal, but that they describe it as dysfunctional. At this point, the therapist may challenge the family description on the basis of his observation. For instance, Mrs. O'Riley came to therapy because of her inability to control her two children, five and three years old. After a half-hour observation of the children's transactions, the therapist cannot detect the elements of incompetence that the mother ascribes to herself in the handling of the children, and he challenges the mother's description of the family. The therapist gives to the mother a variety of tasks that are supposed to test her capacity to control the children, while at the same time he pays attention to the competence of the children and supports their competent maneuvers. Task after task is seen as a sample of the harmonious relationship between the mother and the children.

Unable to convince the therapist of the dysfunctional aspects of the family transaction, Mrs. O'Riley grows increasingly frustrated. This challenge results in her exploring her present relationships with her overly critical divorced husband and her overinvolved critical mother. These relationships reinforce and frame only the dysfunctional aspects of herself; the therapist's framing highlights the more competent parts of herself. This intervention changes the focus of the family away from the mother-child dysfunction. It allows an acknowledgment of the more competent aspects of the mother-child transactions and moves the therapy toward the mother-divorced husband and mother-grandmother holons as a subject for exploration.

Nothing is more irritating and puzzling to family members than a therapist who questions their pathology. They begin to explain themselves and try to convince the therapist about the narrowness of their transactions, only to find in the process of therapy that their operations are far more complex and that aspects of competent and harmonious behavior need to be acknowledged to round out the picture that the family presents.

Statements of puzzled curiosity are ways in which the therapist punctuates his disbelief in the presentation of the family framing. For instance, the therapist may state, "Isn't that extraordinary how you seem to be able to see only one part of your spouse?" or, "Isn't it wonderful how you can elicit from your child only the negative, monsterlike characteristics of him while he seems to present for me only the intelligent and humorous ability to look at life?"

The treatment of the Boyle family is a case in point. This family is made up of the parents, Marion and William, who are in their mid-thirties, and their two children, Joanie, eight, and Dick, five. Marion is a housewife and William owns a small carpentry workshop. They came to therapy because Joanie is underachieving in second grade and acts as if she does not care. They have been seen in four sessions, where they have presented themselves as a well-functioning middle-class American family. William is active in community affairs, and Marion is active in church. They are regarded as an ideal couple.

This is a traditional family with a clearly differentiated gender allocation of roles and functions. Marion, a carefully groomed woman, projects a controlled vitality combined with a coy behavior that frames her as a babydoll. She is the good mother, and the two children are her responsibility; any success or failure by them accrues to her and not to her husband. The children are dressed like small adults ready for Sunday school. Joanie, a blonde like her mother, is already defined as empty-headed, while Dick is defined as competent. William communicates clearly when contacted, but he is mostly quiet, leaving the stage to his wife in this child-centered situation.

In the sessions the family dance is obvious: the spouse holon is patterned on blame and counterblame, followed by withdrawal of the husband and placation by the wife. Marion experiences herself as the ineffective loser in these transactions, but her criticisms have an energy and push that send William into apologies as he withdraws; this is the signal for her to begin her placating movements. The children are friendly, playful, and well behaved. William usually leaves discipline to his wife, but when he takes a position, the children respect it.

In the previous sessions the therapist has been challenging Marion's rather negative view of her relationship to her husband and daughter. He is attracted by Marion's vitality, but he joins William in his request for more participation in the family.

For the third session, the therapist has defined two goals. He will challenge Joanie's "dumb blonde" frame and the spouses' dysfunctional symmetry. The session starts with the children showing off the presents they have brought for the therapist. Dick has used some newly acquired tools to hammer the names SAL and DICK in a wood block; it is really a remarkable piece of workmanship for a five-year-old. Joanie has brought in a stereotyped drawing of a woman with one sad face and one happy face. She has drawn some coins on the top of the page. From the beginning, Minuchin finds himself challenged. He wants to balance his appreciation for Dick's work with an equal support for Joanie's, even though they are of quite different quality.

Minuchin (to Dick, showing his present): Is that for me? May I take it home? What does it say?

Dick: Sal.

Minuchin: That's just great. I love it. You cut that? You are very good with tools. That's great. Now *(turning to Joanie)*, I think that your drawing shows a tremendous amount of cleverness. *(To parents.)* It's not only the esthetics, but Joanie has been working with symbols. Joanie, can you tell me what you did here, because I find that very interesting. What is this face?

Joanie: Somebody mad or sad.

Minuchin: Can you make up a story about that? When I was a kid, I used to make up stories. Make up a story and tell it to your daddy about a person who was mad or sad. *(After a long pause, to father.)* Maybe you can help her.

Joanie: Someone stole Mom's money, then she went to tell the police and Mom got her money back and she's happy again.

Joanie's story is short, undifferentiated, and barely sufficient—the kind of story that children tell to "get by." It is nonetheless syntonic with the family expectation of her capabilities. The problem for the therapist is how to challenge Joanie's limited presentation of herself.

Minuchin: That's the end of the story? Now, make another story about a little child. Make it longer.

Joanie (after a long pause): I lost a puppy and went to a place and cried and told a man to write on a paper that I lost a puppy; and he did and gave it to me. And I went to the city police and they helped me put them on windows and poles and someone had my puppy and they saw the sign for lost puppies and they saw my address on it and phone number and they drove to my house and gave it back to me.

Minuchin: This is a lovely story. You have a great amount of imagination and you put a lot of details there. I didn't know that you could make stories that long and nice. Beautiful!

Mother: I don't really want to make a comment on this, but that was a book that she read once. She gave you a book report on the book she read this year in school.

The therapist feels rather pleased with the "expansion" of Joanie's story and is using it to challenge the parents' narrow expectation of her. He therefore feels cut down by the mother's new information, but resolves to insist on his challenge. In his contact with Joanie during the previous session, he felt pity for her. The narrowness of her constructed "destiny" does not take into account elements of competence that seemed apparent in their contact.

Minuchin (*to mother*): I think that this is you looking at the hole in the doughnut again. This drawing that she did is good for an eight-year-old. (*To Joanie.*) Can you tell us another story? (*After a pause, gives Joanie a drawing she made the previous session.*) Make up a story about this family, one that hasn't been told before. (*Pause.*) Can you help her, Marion?

Mother: Well, I hesitate because you jumped on me about helping her.

Minuchin: Help her in such a way that she does most of the work. That's the important way of helping her.

Mother: How about making a story about a trip with the family. Tell us something special about the trip and about Daddy. What did Daddy do?

Joanie: I have one now! We came to Denver and Daddy was gonna see if he could get a job and went inside an office. This man talked to him and he gave him the job, and when he came out we went to dinner and we celebrated.

Minuchin: That's very nice. Make it a little bit longer.

Joanie: And then we went home and had presents for him and opened them up and he had something he always wanted and it was a wrist watch, and he wore it until it got rusty and he shined it up, and when Dick grew up to wear it, he gave it to Dick. The next day after Dick got the wrist watch, we went on a walk and came to a meadow of flowers and Dick picked me a bouquet of flowers.

Minuchin: That's a very lovely story, and I like that very much. Marion, she didn't read that any place?

Mother: No, she didn't read that anywhere.

Minuchin: Can you see the doughnut?

Mother: Yes, I have a very nice doughnut. I don't see any holes there.

The therapist's higher expectation of Joanie's capacity creates a resonant field in which Joanie uses herself differently. In the therapist-child holon, Joanie responds to different rules and expands her repertoire. The therapeutic problem then becomes the support of alternative transactions in the larger family holon. The session continues with Dick telling a story of his own, and then the children put on a puppet show that they prepared at home while the parents and the therapist sit as appreciative audience. During this part of the session the therapist congratulates the parents for the success they have had in raising such exploratory and creative children. The children are then asked to leave, and the session focuses on the couple.

Minuchin (*to wife*): Why do you think he's not around?

Wife: Well, I think Will is a workaholic. He is consumed by work. He thinks about it constantly. When we go to bed at night, he lies there with a scratch pad drawing pictures of what he's going to do tomorrow.

Minuchin: Marion, what should the wife of a workaholic do to change him?

Wife: I suppose I should become aggressive. I am not an aggressive person, but I guess I should become a temptress and throw myself at him every time I get the opportunity and take his mind off of his work.

Minuchin: Ask him if that would be helpful?

Wife: Would that be helpful, Will?

Husband: It certainly would, because in a lot of ways work throws itself at me in the form of telephone calls and responsibility. It's the same kind of thing.

Minuchin: I think there is something that Will is not telling you because he doesn't know it. In some way or other, when he comes home, he is younger than when he's at work. He feels more like a competent adult when he's working. Can you check to see if that is true?

Wife: Is that right? Do you feel that way?

Husband: I know that the way I interact with the guys at work and with customers is really different from when I'm acting at home. They're expecting from me different behavior from your expectation at home.

Minuchin: He said that when he is away from home, he feels competent and responsible and committed. I heard you say last session that you would like him to be committed and responsible at home. How is it that he has these capacities outside and when he comes home, he becomes defensive, apologetic, dependent, guilty, and not very giving?

Wife: I'd like to know why. What triggers that change?

Minuchin: He is outside, the kind of man—

Wife: That I want him to be at home.

The therapist is working from a theoretical schema that the rules of this spouse holon control the behavior of its members in ways that make them less competent than in their extrafamilial functioning. He introduces this construction, focused on the husband's constrained functioning at home, to use as a lever in changing the spouses' way of legitimizing their behavior.

Wife: I find it difficult to believe him if he says he's going to do something in the house. He's going to build in new kitchen cabinets, but I've lived with him for seven years and I've seen hundreds of projects begun at home and I haven't seen anything finished.

Minuchin: If he's such a competent man and you want a kitchen cabinet and that is something he does very well and he has not done it in seven years, you are a failure.

By suggesting that the husband's work at home is a measure of his response to the wife, the therapist, working with the complementarity of spouses, opens up for the wife the possibility of changing the husband's behavior. By choosing the kitchen cabinet as a concrete metaphor of the couple's relationship, the therapist facilitates, in a therapy of action, a fast movement toward experimenting with alternatives.

Minuchin: You need to change him, Marion. This man that is an expert creative constructor of things has a home where, for seven years, he has not made a kitchen where he can say, "I am very pleased with what I have done." And he didn't do it because he doesn't want to give you something. Why doesn't he want to give you something?

Wife (to husband): Do you think I'm selfish? Do you think I spend more time being concerned about myself than others?

Husband: My impulse answer is yes.

Wife: I think you're right. I'm just turning into a self-centered person.

Minuchin: Marion, I am interested in the fact that this man does not want to give you a kitchen. Didn't you realize that?

Wife: No, because he always manages to make it seem like he doesn't have time.

Minuchin: He gave the time to somebody else. He just organizes it so that he doesn't give it to you.

The wife's offering of her "selfishness" as an explanation for their transactions is a homeostatic maneuver. The therapist avoids "fairness" and continues pushing her to demand from her husband a concrete change in his functioning at home.

Husband: A key to this might be the day that I put in the French doors in the living room and one of my main carpenters told me that he didn't want to come back and work anymore at the house. He just couldn't work around you. And I have thought that I have trouble, too; whenever I'm working, I can't work in the same room with you. But I can't really tell you why—some dynamics of our interactions that causes me to be inefficient and causes me not to want to accomplish very much. And the reason that comes to mind is that you aren't supporting me and you're not agreeing with what I'm doing. You're not accepting it.

Minuchin: Can you change your wife so that you can build things for both of you? This kitchen cabinet is a symbol of your marriage; you just have not married yet. Do you want to be married to your wife?

Will offers his "dynamics" as an explanation of the homeostatic rut that controls the spouse holon. The therapist avoids a therapy of understanding deficits and keeps the focus on the construction of the kitchen cabinet as a metaphor of changing the marriage.

Minuchin: You will need to change her so that you can be married to her. Because the way in which you are relating to her now is to escape from her whenever she needs you. Marion, do you want to be married to him? Do you really want to be married to him?

Wife: Yes, I do.

Minuchin: Then you will need to change him so that he's at home, responsible and committed as he is in other situations. You will need to change this man if you want to stay married to him.

Wife: That will be a hard one.

Minuchin: Don't let it be. I'm going through the ritual of marrying you. I am saying to you, "Change each other so that you can become a couple." And then, Will, you will build this kitchen cabinet, but not for her. For both of you. How is it you don't feel like that is your kitchen as well?

Husband: She told me it wasn't my kitchen.

Wife: I think the reason I told you that it was my kitchen would be the same reason you would tell me that your workshop is your workshop.

Minuchin (to both): Are you married?

Husband: Yes, I think we are.

Wife: What do you feel like when you visit me in my kitchen every morning, when you come in and eat breakfast?

Husband: I hesitate to say every morning, but as a general rule I don't feel as comfortable a lot of time.

Minuchin (to both): You have a task, the task is to build a kitchen that is for both of you. It is a place that you build together. And Will, it's not only your business; it's the business of both of you.

Wife (to husband): Oh, but you made it very clear to me on many occasions that it's your business.

Minuchin: Of course, because you're not yet married. But when you become married, it will become your business as well. Will, do you want this woman to be your wife?

Husband: I do.

Minuchin: Do you want to build a kitchen for her and for you?

Husband: I certainly do.

Minuchin: Marion, do you want this man for your husband?

Wife: Yes, I do.

Minuchin: Do you want to help him in his business?

Wife: Yes.

Husband: The thing that comes to my mind as we're doing this discussion is that we should remap the plans and make a schedule and just plan to do the kitchen all the way through. *(To wife.)* Would you like that?

Wife: Yeah, when are we going to do it?

Husband: Start it today. I think what we should do is build the kitchen and try to develop the interaction pattern that makes us work together, and we should have another symbolic marriage ceremony and start all over again.

The last part of the session takes the form of a marriage ceremony in which the therapist qua healer performs the ritual of recommitment to a changed spouse holon.

This is the end of a road along which therapeutic techniques have been displayed. There are, of course, many other techniques that we do not use but which serve well in the hands of experienced therapists. But technique is not the goal. The goal can be achieved only by putting aside technique.

18 Beyond Technique

After years of painstaking attention to the finest details of the techniques of martial art, the samurai had become a craftsman. He knew the proper shouting, how to distract and parry, when to use the heavy sword for two arms, and what step to choose for the final thrust. Still, he was not satisfied. What if he used the proper techniques in the wrong situations? What if he used the sword for his own aggrandizement?

Tradition told him that he was too close to his trade. The sword was still a sword, not yet an extension of his arm. So with the appropriate ceremony, he put aside his trade and went in search of esthetics, harmony, and distance, so that ultimately he and the sword would be one. This chapter is that kind of ceremony. It is a valedictory for the techniques of family therapy, so that the reader can put them aside, and go in search of wisdom.

Over the years, Minuchin has collected anecdotes, thoughts, and fables on the techniques of family therapy, pro and con. Carl Whitaker tells the story of the strategy of bottle feeding patients. One day in his office, a mother left her infant's bottle. When the next patient commented on it, Whitaker offered him the bottle. From then on, bottle feeding became an important technique in the weaponry of his team of therapists, who encouraged their patients to regress, using the bottle as a prop. The therapists were full of excitement, and so were the sessions. Patients brought meaningful associations, and therapy achieved new dimensions. For a while, it seemed that The Technique had been found.

But with the passage of time, the excitement wore off. Patients and therapists became less enthusiastic, and ultimately bored. Finally milk became not a pathway, but plain milk.

By then, arm wrestling had been introduced in the team, and for a while, it seemed that The Technique had again been found. But with the passage of time, arm wrestling too became not a pathway, but only a way of finding out whose arm was stronger. The point, according to Whitaker, is that each technique was useful as long as it produced excitement and curiosity in the therapist. Like the Wizard of Oz's medal, which gave courage only to the courageous, technique is only a vehicle for the therapist's creative exploration.[1]

Frank Pittman is another therapist who seemed to have discovered The Technique, when he lighted on the technique of the small wet poodle. He was conducting a home visit on a rainy day. In the middle of the session, the husband left, and the psychotic wife stiffened. Her face went blank, her eyes glazed, and she fell to the floor. After a quick examination to ensure that his patient was physically all right, Pittman tried a series of ingenious, but unsuccessful, maneuvers to bring his patient out of her catatonia to her previous, more manageable psychotic state. Suddenly he heard a frantic scratching at the kitchen door. He opened it, and a small wet spaniel ran into the room. He shook himself, liberally anointing his mistress and the floor, and then jumped on her, anxiously licking her face. The woman sat up and launched into a tirade, roundly scolding the spaniel for wetting her good rug. The only drawback to this most remarkable technique, according to Pittman, is that so few cases can be found with the appropriate elements for its utilization. Would that every catatonic woman had a best rug and a small wet spaniel.[2]

Chloe Madanes has an endless capacity for tailoring techniques to specific family situations. She tells of working with one case in which a pediatrician referred an 11-year-old diabetic girl who was not responding to pediatric management. Her mother, a woman in her late thirties, was also a diabetic. She appeared in more need of care than the child. The family was on welfare, and the mother did not take proper care of her illness or the child's. Thinking on her feet, Madanes asked a nurse who was observing the session to lend her white tunic to the mother. The mother was asked to pretend that she was a nurse obeying the therapist's instructions in the care of her daughter. At the next session, Madanes came prepared with a small white uniform for the daughter and initiated a pretending game in which the daughter nursed the mother. Inducing a series of changes in the mother-daughter holon by this maneuver, Madanes was soon successful in changing the pattern of diabetic management in both patients. Unfortunately, this technique too is one for which very few families are suited. It is now a strategy without a patient.[3]

Milton Erickson is well known for his ingenious techniques. One of his patients was a psychotic who thought he was Christ. "I hear you are a carpenter," Erickson said. "Will you help me build some shelves?" Another time he told a mother to sit on her impossible young child until the appropriate hierarchy was defined. He warned the mother to prepare for a long siege and gave her specific instructions to gather books, food, and her knitting.[4]

Although Erickson's techniques are funny, unusual, and as magical as the work of a sorcerer, his videotaped sessions are still impressive for the warmth of his voice and the poetic quality of his descriptions; he was more like a wise and loving uncle than a magician. A week before he died, I met him, and was rewarded by an encounter with a truly remarkable man. He told me that in late adolescence he had contracted poliomyelitis. Almost paralyzed, he asked his mother to put a mirror high on the wall so he could observe the goings on in the house. He spent a lot of time watching his infant sister learning how to walk and following in vivid detail all the movements a toddler uses to stand up in her crib: extending her arms, flexing her fingers to grasp the bars, stretching her body, rearranging her feet—all the movements that an adult does automatically. He thought then that since he must have learned all of these complicated operations as an infant, he would not have to learn how to get up. He had only to remember.

Out of these operations, Erickson developed a hopeful conceptualization of the possibilities inherent in human nature. He was convinced that people, given the proper context, could stretch, expand, and recover lost skills. His techniques were built on this basis: diverse forms embedded in a matrix of optimism.

When Edgar Auerswald, Charles H. King, Braulio Montalvo, Clara Rabinowitz, and I began working with families of delinquent inner-city children at the Wiltwyck School for Boys, the only source for techniques of family therapy was one article by Don Jackson. We used a one-way mirror to observe each other and learn from our own mistakes. In those days our mode of treatment was confrontative; we were going to save the family from the world and from themselves. Out of this pitting of the therapist's determination and optimism against the family's more informed hopelessness, a transformation frequently occurred: the families accommodated to the therapist's insistence that alternatives were available. I now doubt the wisdom of the techniques we used, but I am certain that the therapists' zeal and commitment were helpful. How long the transformations lasted against the realities of racial and economic oppression, I am not certain. I know that in some cases the help was lasting; in others, the realities of the slum proved much stronger than the therapeutic constructions.[5]

Over time, a number of changes were made in our approach, some theoretical, others methodological, and there were also changes in the way of describing our work. In the early period of family therapy, the efficacy of this radically different approach to conceptualization and treatment had to be proved to the psychoanalytic establishment and to ourelves. Our descriptions of therapy included what now seems an unncessary bravado. In our challenge to the field, operations that seemed too supportive, interpretive, or even humanistic were played down, and our differences with traditional psychodynamic theory were emphasized. Today, when explorations of similarities are no longer taboo, our descriptions are fuller. Other techniques have evolved, many of which utilize the wisdom of techniques we once attacked. Time, experience, and acceptance have made our descriptions of therapy less shrill. Our techniques encompass more, and are increasingly varied.

In my own case, my style has grown softer, and more effective. I feel free to use compassion and humor in joining with families. I have learned to use my life experience and my fellow feeling for families as part of the therapeutic process. Having made my share of mistakes in my life, I don't expect my patients to be perfect. I know that family members do the best they can, and that sometimes the results are very destructive. I am supportive, because I know that I cannot find a wrinkle in any patient's psyche that has not already been pinpointed, examined, and magnified by that person and by every family member. My challenges are sharper and clearer, and at the same time I have learned how to encourage the exploration of alternatives.

All in all, I do the same things better with less effort, enjoying it more, like Maurice Chevalier, who could sum up all the charm and skill of his younger days in the way he moved his straw hat. I am less judgmental and more demanding. I can allow myself to enjoy my creativity and vanity. With the acceptance of both my skills and my limitations, my range of effectiveness has increased. "The road is how you walk it," and by now, the traveling and the traveler are one.[6]

Close this book now. It is a book on techniques. Beyond technique, there is the widom which is knowledge of the interconnectedness of things. "Wisdom," Gregory Bateson says, "demands not only a recognition of the facts of circuitry, but a conscious recognition, rooted in both intellectual and emotional experience, synthesizing the two."[7] When techniques are guided by such wisdom, then therapy becomes healing.

Notes
Case Index
General Index

Notes

1. SPONTANEITY

1. Miyamoto Musashi, *A Book of Five Rings: A Guide to Strategy*, trans. Victor Harris (Woodstock, N.Y.: The Overlook Press, 1974), pp. 78–79.

2. Jay Haley, *Problem Solving Therapy* (San Francisco: Jossey-Bass, 1976), p. 172.

2. FAMILIES

Epigraph: Lewis Thomas, *The Lives of a Cell: Notes of a Biology Watcher* (New York: Bantam Books, 1974), p. 147.

1. Salvador Minuchin, Bernice L. Rosman, and Lester Baker, *Psychosomatic Families: Anorexia Nervosa in Context* (Cambridge: Harvard University Press, 1978), p. 45.

2. Albert Scheflen, "Family Communication and Social Connectedness in the Development of Schizophrenia," in Maurizio Andolfi and Israel Zwerling, *Dimensions in Family Therapy* (New York: Guilford Press, 1980), chap. 9.

3. Arthur Koestler, *Janus: A Summing Up* (New York: Vintage Books, 1979), p. 33.

4. Murray Bowen, *Family Therapy in Clinical Practice* (New York: Jason Aronson, 1978), pp. 306–307.

5. P. Glansdorff and Ilya Prigogine, *Thermodynamic Theory of Structure, Stability and Fluctuations* (New York: Wiley, 1971), pp. xiv–xxi.

6. Erich Jantsch, *Design for Evolution: Self Organization and Planning in the Life of Human Systems* (New York: George Braziller, 1975), p. 37. The authors are indebted to Paul F. Dell and Harold A. Goolishian, whose paper "Order Through Fluctuation: An Evolutionary Epistemology for Human Systems" (presented at the Annual Scientific Meeting of the A. K. Rice Institute, Houston, Texas, 1979) enhanced our interpretation of Prigogine and Jantsch.

3. JOINING

1. Donald Meltzer, "Routine and Inspired Interpretations," *Contemporary Psychoanalysis* 14, no. 2 (April 1978): 211–225.
2. Lyman Wynne, I. Ryckoff, J. Day, and S. Hersch, "Pseudo-Mutuality in the Family Relationships of Schizophrenics," *Psychiatry* 21 (1958): 205–220.
3. Jay Haley and Lynn Hoffman, *Techniques of Family Therapy* (New York: Basic Books, 1967), pp. 307–308; Augustus Y. Napier with Carl A. Whitaker, *The Family Crucible* (New York: Harper & Row, 1978), p. 9.
4. Mara Selvini-Palazzoli, L. Boscolo, G. Cecchin, and G. Prata, *Paradox and Counter Paradox* (New York: Jason Aronson, 1978).
5. Murray Bowen, *Family Therapy in Clinical Practice* (New York: Jason Aronson, 1978), p. 310.
6. Dorothy R. Blitsten, *The Social Theories of Harry Stack Sullivan* (New York: William-Frederick Press, 1953).

4. PLANNING

1. Hope J. Leichter and William E. Mitchell, *Kinship and Casework* (New York: Russell Sage Foundation, 1967).
2. Salvador Minuchin, Braulio Montalvo, B. G. Guerney, Jr., B. L. Rosman, and Florence Schumer, *Families of the Slums* (New York: Basic Books, 1967).
3. Minuchin et al., *Families of the Slums.*

5. CHANGE

1. Augustus Y. Napier with Carl A. Whitaker, *The Family Crucible* (New York: Harper & Row, 1978); Cloe Madanes and Jay Haley, "Dimensions of Family Therapy," *Journal of Mental and Nervous Diseases* 165, no. 2 (1977): 88–98.
2. Salvador Minuchin, Bernice L. Rosman, and Lester Baker, *Psychosomatic Families: Anorexia Nervosa in Context* (Cambridge: Harvard University Press, 1978), chap. 9.

7. ENACTMENT

Epigraph: William B. Yeats, "Among School Children," in *The New Oxford Book of English Verse, 1250–1950,* ed. Helen Gardner (New York: Oxford University Press, 1972), pp. 824–826.

1. Henry Bergson, *An Introduction to Metaphysics,* trans. T. E. Hulme (New York: Liberal Arts Press, 1955).

8. FOCUS

1. Videotape, "Heroin My Baby," ed. Jay Haley.

10. RESTRUCTURING

1. Herbert A. Simon, "The Architecture of Complexity," *Proceedings of the American Philosophical Society* 106, no. 6 (December 1962).
2. Peter L. Berger and Thomas Luckmann, *The Social Construction of Reality* (New York: Doubleday, 1967) pp. 53–59, 118.
3. Murray Bowen, *Family Therapy in Clinical Practice* (New York: Jason Aronson, 1978) p. 530.

13. COMPLEMENTARITY

1. *The I Ching or Book of Changes,* trans. Cary F. Baynes and Richard Wilhelm (Princeton, N.J.: Princeton University Press, 1967), p. 570.

2. Lewis Thomas, *The Lives of a Cell: Notes of a Biology Watcher* (New York: Bantam Books, 1974), p. 167.

3. Fritjof Capra, *The Tao of Physics* (Boulder: Shambhala, 1975), pp. 151–160.

4. Thomas, *Lives of a Cell,* p. 12.

5. Lama Angarika Govinda, "Logic and Symbol in the Multi-Dimensional Conception of the Universe," in *Main Currents,* vol. 25, p. 60.

6. Salvador Minuchin, *Families and Family Therapy* (Cambridge: Harvard University Press, 1974), p. 159.

7. Ernst F. Schumacher, *Small Is Beautiful* (New York: Harper & Row, 1973), pg. 14.

14. REALITIES

1. Richard Llewellyn, *A Man in a Mirror* (Garden City, N.Y.: Doubleday, 1961).

2. Sol Worth and John Adair, "The Navajo as a Filmmaker: A Brief Report of Some Recent Research in the Cross-Cultural Aspects of Film Communication," in *American Anthropology* 69 (1967): 76–78.

3. Richard Chalfen and Jay Haley, "Reaction to Socio-Documentary Film Research in a Mental Health Clinic," in *American Journal of Orthopsychiatry* 41, no. 1 (January 1971): 91–100.

4. Jose Ortega y Gasset, *Meditations on Don Quixote* (New York: W. W. Norton, 1961), p. 87.

5. George Herbert Mead, *On Social Psychology* (Chicago: University of Chicago Press, 1977), pp. 202, 207.

6. Dorothy R. Blitsten, *The Social Theories of Harry Stack Sullivan* (New York: William-Frederick Press, 1953), p. 138.

7. Peter Berger and Thomas Luckmann, *The Social Construction of Reality* (New York: Doubleday, 1967), pp. 94–95.

8. Berger and Luckmann, *Social Construction of Reality,* p. 125.

9. Nigel Dennis, *Cards of Identity* (New York: Vanguard Press, 1955), p. 118.

15. CONSTRUCTIONS

1. Ivan Boszormenyi-Nagy, "Contextual Therapy: Therapeutic Leverages in Mobilizing Trust," in *The American Family,* Unit IV, no. 2 (Philadelphia: Smith, Kline, & French, 1979).

2. Jose Ortega y Gasset, *Meditations on Don Quixote* (New York: W. W. Norton, 1961), p. 184.

16. PARADOXES

1. Rohrbaugh, Tennen et al., "Paradoxical Strategies in Psychotherapy," Paper read at meeting of the American Psychological Association, San Francisco, 1977.

2. Michel Foucault, *Madness and Civilization: A History of Insanity in the Age of Reason* (New York: Pantheon, 1965).

3. Carlos Castenada, *A Journey to Ixtlan* (New York: Simon & Schuster, 1973), p. xi.

17. STRENGTHS

1. Jane Howard, *Families* (New York: Berkley Books, 1980), p. 58.

2. Philip Larkin, "This Be The Verse," in *High Windows* (London: Faber and Faber, 1974), p. 30.

3. R. D. Laing, *Facts of Life* (New York: Ballantine Books, 1976), pp. 2, 3.

4. Andrew Ferber, Marilyn Mendelsohn, and Augustine Napier, *The Book of Family Therapy* (Boston: Houghton Mifflin, 1972), pp. 90–91.

5. Howard, *Families,* pp. 112–113.

6. John E. Bell, *The Family in the Hospital: Lessons from Developing Countries* (Chevy Chase, Md.: NIMH, 1969), pp. 3–6.

7. Betty McDonald, *Anybody Can Do Anything* (New York: J. B. Lippincott, 1950), p. 11.

18. BEYOND TECHNIQUE

1. Carl A. Whitaker and D. V. Keith, "Experiential/Symbolic Family Therapy," in *Handbook of Family Therapy* (New York: Brunner/Mazel, in press).

2. Andrew Ferber, Marilyn Mendelsohn, and Augustus Napier, *The Book of Family Therapy* (Boston: Houghton Mifflin, 1972), p. 588.

3. Personal communications with Cloe Madanes.

4. Jay Haley, *Uncommon Therapy: The Psychiatric Techniques of Milton H. Erickson, M.D.* (New York: W. W. Norton, 1973), pg. 214, 290.

5. Salvador Minuchin, Bravlio Montalvo, B. G. Guerney, Jr., B. L. Rosman, and Florence Schumer, *Families of the Slums* (New York: Basic Books, 1967).

6. Salvador Minuchin, *Familias y Terapia Familiar* (Barcelona: Granica Editor, 1977), p. 178.

7. Mary Catherine Bateson, "Daddy, Can a Scientist Be Wise?" in *About Bateson: An Introduction to Gregory Bateson,* ed. John Brockman, (New York: E. P. Dutton, 1977), p. 69.

Case Index

General Index